WHAT N(

Sees

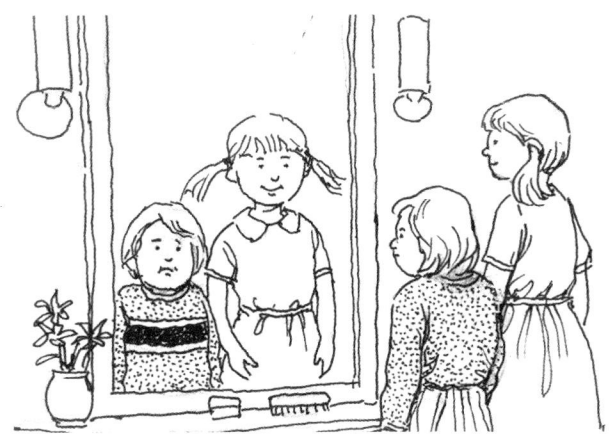

Anne-Pia Nygård

Translated from the Norwegian by
Tracy and Tim Rishton

Loaghtan Books
17 Onslow Avenue
Sutton
Surrey
SM2 7ED

Typesetting and origination by
Loaghtan Books

Printed and bound by
Lavenham Press Ltd

Published by Loaghtan Books

ISBN: 978 1 908060 04 4

www.loaghtanbooks.com

First published in English: September 2012

Front cover: Anne-Pia with her father in Sophies Minde Orthopaedic Hospital, being 'stretched'

Rear cover: Anne-Pia aloft in the *Lord Nelson*

Title page: Anne-Pia realising sadly that she is different from her friends

CONTENTS

ACKNOWLEDGEMENTS

Thank you

Gus for your ideas and for your everyday inspiration. I love you
Mum and dad, my brothers and sisters, for your love and support
Uncle Harald for your wonderful drawings
Tim and Tracy for believing in my project
Sara for making it come true

Anne-Pia Nygård

ANNE-PIA'S NORWAY

The outline map below is intended only to give a rough idea of the location of some of the places mentioned in the text. The map shows many of the places important to Anne-Pia within Norway; it does not cover her life in Denmark or her visits to other parts of Europe.

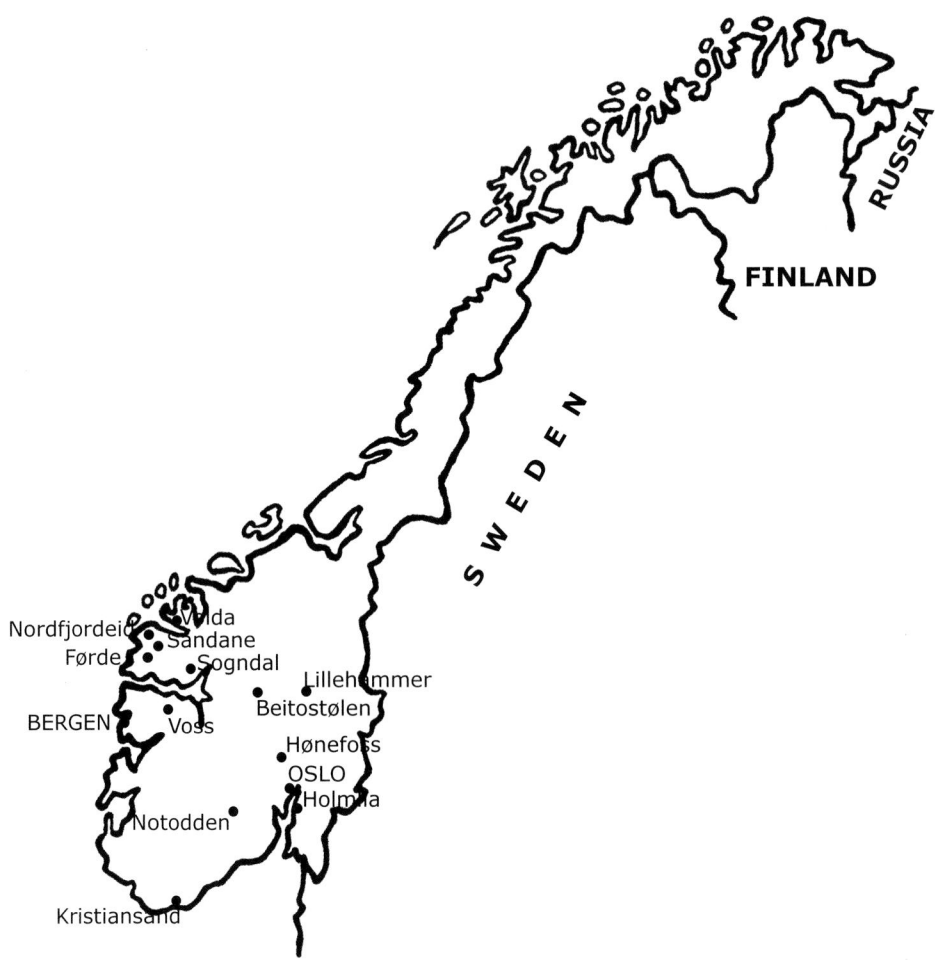

I don't remember it.

I try to look back, but I can't find my way back to exactly that point. To when I could no longer walk.

The changes were gradual, but even so there was a certain point when it happened.

9 January 1988. One minute I was on my feet, the next minute I couldn't get out of the bean bag.

It is odd. I can easily remember things that happened before, and I can easily remember things that happened after. But just that moment?

I don't know what went through my head in the seconds that it took. Maybe it was minutes. Did my thoughts gallop away, like life flashes before the eyes of someone who is dying, or was my mind empty as I sat there and life ebbed out of my legs? 'It's OK, Dad, I knew this would happen'. He tells me that's what I said. I don't remember. I was surprisingly at ease with my new situation. Calm. More so than my parents. But that's the way it is. It is always more difficult for those who have to watch. We don't talk about what's happened. I don't talk about it to them or to anyone else. They don't talk about it with me. Maybe they didn't think I needed to talk. That's true. In the beginning it was just a relief not to have to walk. Not to need to use my tired legs any more. But after living with the consequences for a while it was different. What had actually happened? By the time I had got to that point, everyone was used to the new situation, and saw how well I tackled it. I couldn't then start saying: 'By the way, I am not coping with this very well after all!'

What is a normal reaction to something that hasn't happened to you before? There was no pain to deal with. There was no dramatic car crash to wake screaming in the night at the memory of.

There was – nothing really. And yet enough that the life I knew had disappeared and another taken its place.

It started long ago, the reason that my legs became lame. I suppose it really started before I was born. Perhaps it didn't need to have been like that, but it was.

I am trying to work out how what has happened to me has affected me. It is not always actual situations that I remember. It may be just a feeling. I recognise a smell, and a memory associated with it pops into my mind. A waft of perfume mixed with cigarette smoke and I am right back to the orthopaedic hospital, Sophies Minde. The waft of smoked fish and boiled carrots from an extractor fan and I am waiting for the food trolley to get to room 210. The day's high-point. A tin cup, an orange plastic tray, and a glass of squash, a long white straw packed in easy-rip paper packaging. 'Can I have some more?' 'And more squash?' 'Can I take a straw?' and then 'puff', the high-point is over. Quarter of an hour is all it took. Twenty-three hours and forty-five minutes until next time. But there is supper and breakfast in between, I suppose.

I'll rewind a bit. We'll return here later.

Birth. Those nine months before I was born. What went wrong?

There are medical terms but no answers, just questions. 'These things happen.' 'It's a rare case.' 'I am sure there is someone who knows what we can do.' Reams of headed note paper: *Dear Colleague, I enclose the case notes and X-rays of patient born on… in the year… Could you give your medical opinion… Possible further investigation with you?… With grateful thanks.*

My birth and the nine months leading up to it are impossible to remember, at any rate. I have gone back. I have a memory of remembering the point, I just don't know if it is a real memory of what actually happened, even though I know it must have happened because I'm here!

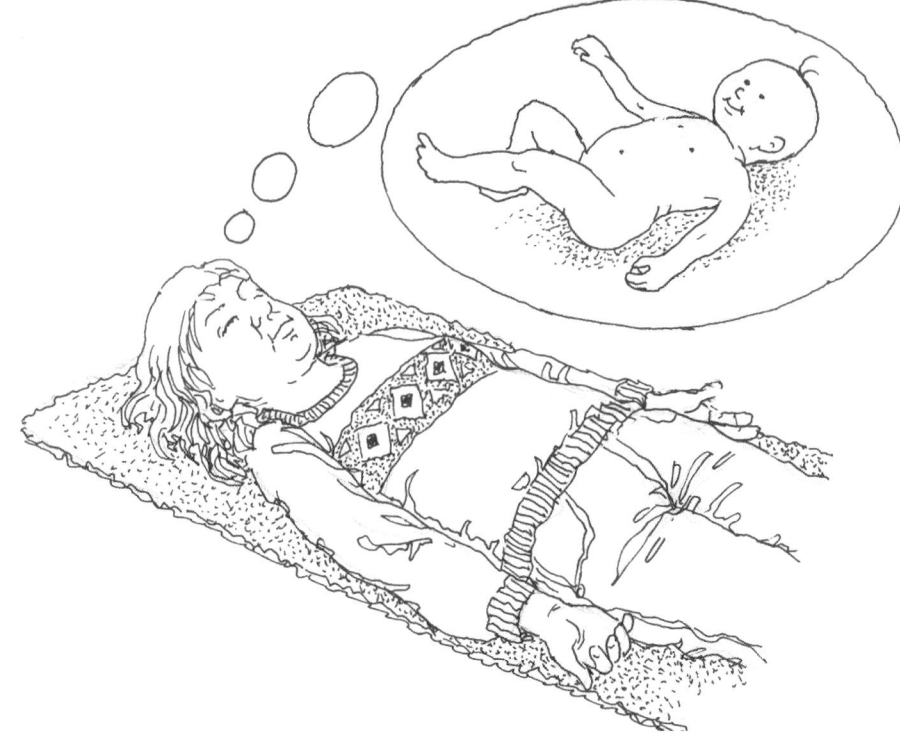

REGRESSION

I can see myself from above… it's a bit unclear to begin with but then it gets clearer and clearer. I eventually focus, focus in on myself. I am in my body at the same time as looking at myself from above. It is a huge shock to see what my body has become. As well as being wrinkly and red, my upper body is kind of squashed up at the top. It is worse than I expected and I feel more alone than ever.

We are lying on red mats on the floor. Our heads in the centre of the circle formed by our bodies. Ten warm bodies breathing the way we are being told. Breathe calm and deep, and then fast until you get inside yourself. Relax. Listen to my voice. I am with you the whole time.

Rune goes round in the middle taking time for each of us. Touching us gently with his fingertips if he sees we need someone.

I have been to the meditation group before, but this is the first time I've done anything like this. At the beginning of the course we had to say why we'd come and what expectations we had.

'What was your birth like?' asked Rune when I told the group that I felt like I wasn't getting anywhere in life.

'What?' I was bowled over by the question and could not imagine what that had to do with anything.

'Was it a difficult birth? When we feel that things have ground to a halt we can often trace it back to our birth.'

'Well, I don't know.' And I truly didn't. 'I was born with damage to my back, but I don't know anything about the actual birth.'

We jump forward in time. Again I feel alone. I am in hospital far from Mum and Dad. I don't see anything. I feel. I am sad because they aren't there. I understand but at the same time don't understand why they can't be there. I am all on my own and the only thing I want to do is cry.

She will soon be a Mum again. He will be a Dad again. Paul will be a big brother.

She is about to give birth, to push her into the world. Earlier in the pregnancy Mum thought there was something wrong. Stomach cramps that wouldn't stop. The doctor wouldn't even test a urine sample from his patient. 'I will write a prescription for some tablets, they will sort it out.' Mum tried to put aside the unpleasant memory of the doctor.

As a paediatric nurse she was taught that the doctor is always right. On the maternity unit they had to have all the babies lined up ready when the doctor made his rounds. You did not speak unless spoken to by the doctor. The atmosphere was always different when he was in the room. People held their breath for fear of doing or saying something wrong. The doctor moved from baby to baby as the nurses stood to attention.

She tried to reassure herself that he was a doctor, he knew best, but when Christmas came and went the pain was still there. She decided to seek a second opinion. It is in the new doctor's surgery that she is told. That she is pregnant. A smile creeps across her mouth before the next thought comes.

'The tablets?' She knows how vulnerable an unborn baby is.

'You should never have been given those.'

The doctor's brow is wrinkled. She is tight-lipped, which causes her lips to appear through her lipstick her and there. Before she hears the words Mum knows what the doctor is going to say. Her subconscious has known it all along. Now as she hears the words she tries to focus on the name badge on the doctor's white coat but she has no idea what it says. Whether it is a short name or a long name, or whether she can see the name badge at all.

The room slowly starts to spin.

Mum moves her gaze to the blood-pressure measure on the table in front of her. She suddenly can't remember what it is used for. She feels sick. Is it morning sickness this late in the day? Is she spinning or is it just her head? Why else would she be sitting there hanging on to her own arm? Hugging herself as if to protect the life she now knows lives within her.

The complete joy stolen from this mother and father. They have been thrown defenceless to the ground by a doctor who soon will be sued by another woman. They feel happiness begin to emerge, to stir into being, only to be swept away by grief when they least expect it. When they allow themselves to dream about their new little boy or girl. Who will he or she look like? What will this child be good at? Will he or she have blonde curls like Paul or be dark-haired like both parents? It's just at moments like these that grief creeps up and swallows them in doubts.

We wanted a brother or sister for Paul. We will be grateful if the child lives and is healthy. We won't spoil everything with any other wish.

They have been looking forward to a new baby but, behind the smiles they gave to the people who wanted to chat about the big event, there lay the unease of not knowing whether something had gone wrong. What do you say to family members when this should be such a happy time? What might the response be? Should family and friends be happy or should they only show sympathy and concern? Not least, can they talk to each other about their thoughts and feelings?

This was before the use of ultrasound scans so they knew nothing about this unborn baby. The new doctor tried to comfort the parents: 'the baby has a very strong heartbeat; all the signs are that this is a normal pregnancy.'

This is my life before I am born; I am already a misdiagnosed patient. It rarely happens, but it happened to me. Who knows if this is how it was meant to be, but this is how it was.

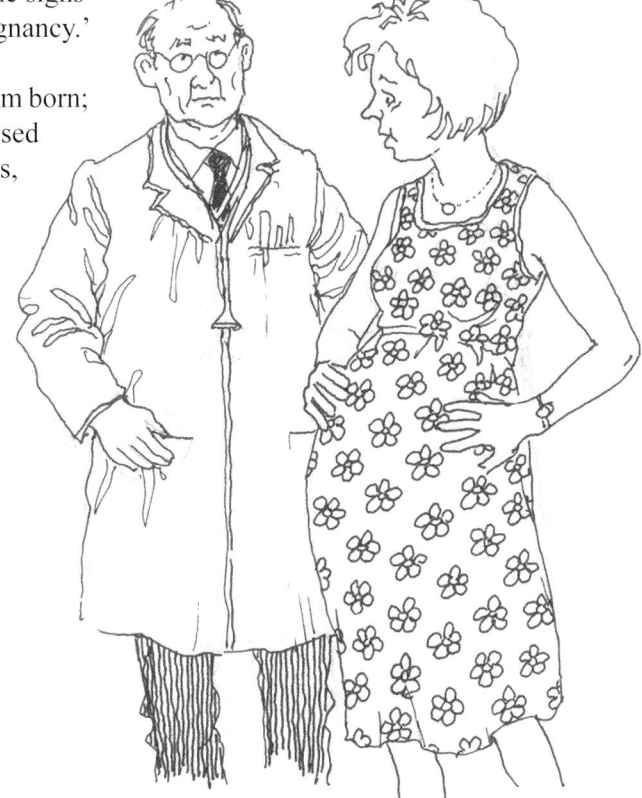

The calendar shows 10 August 1977. The pregnancy was normal. The birth goes smoothly. Flat nose and wrinkly skin. On her head is a mane of black hair making a striking contrast to her bright red face. Granddad takes a look and says she looks like a piglet.

For one day they are allowed to be happy before grief hits back. This time, too, the messenger is wearing a uniform. They thought the battle was over, that all their fears were groundless. It is the day after the birth and nobody is visiting. Dad is back at work. Paul is with his grandparents. The rhythm is just getting going. A midwife, a group of midwives approach Mum's bed.

'Has the doctor been to speak to you?'

'No?…'

'I don't suppose he has had time. I might as well tell you then, did you see that there was something wrong with the baby?'

Mum hesitates. At the women's clinic she had seen many newborns with a look of Down's Syndrome, and it was one of the first things she looked for in her own babies. She had not seen anything like that in her own and does not know what the midwife is getting at.

'She did seem a bit squashed,' says Mum carefully, 'but not all new-borns are beautiful immediately…'

'The baby has no neck,' continues the midwife, 'and she has a curvature of the spine. She has been born with something called Kyphoscoliosis.'

Mum is afraid as the midwife stands over her and explains. Tomorrow Dad will be at her parents to celebrate Paul's third birthday. Since they haven't yet got a telephone in their flat she will have to wait until he's there to tell him.

Dad leaves the party and comes straight to the hospital. Soon after, the paediatrician confirms the diagnosis and explains that they cannot do anything with it yet. The doctor says that all they can do is wait.

Kyphosis is a backwards curvature of the upper spine. Scoliosis is a crooked back. More correctly, it is a sideways curvature of the spine. It is usually teenage girls who develop spinal scoliosis. The crooked back develops and they have to strengthen the spine with exercise or use a corset to straighten it.

It is very unusual to be born with scoliosis, and the reason for this congenital vertebral anomaly is unknown, but early embryonic damage is a possible cause. That is when the foetus is in its fifth to eighth week of development.

Scoliosis is treated with a corset when the curvature of the spine is over thirty degrees. In 460 BC, Hippocrates, the father of medicine, was using splint corsets. In Paris in 1582 the surgeon Ambroise Paré was treating people with iron corsets. Advanced corsets were developed in Germany three hundred years later.

In 1911 Russel Hibbs attempted the first spinal operation. The operation took place at New York's orthopaedic hospital but post-operative complications gave him a bad reputation.

In 1946 Blount and Schmidt developed the Milwaukee Corset for the treatment of scoliosis and kyphosis. This corset has been developed today incorporating various improvements including the Boston Corset.

Regarding surgery (which is considered when the curvature of the spine is over forty-five degrees) the Harrington staves were used during the 1960s. Since then, various staves/screws and rods have been used. Harrington staves were used until the end of the 1980s. Cotrel and Dubousset developed (CD) instrumentation in 1988; a twin-stave system attached in several places to the spine by means either of hooks or screws. The Harrington technique works well on the whole; small neurological complications occur in one per cent of patients.

Total paralysis (paraplegia) is a rare complication.

Ancient carvings have been found showing curvature of the spine.

Due to the situation, they were able to bring their daughter home from the hospital early.

'I hope to see you at Sandane', says the midwife. Everything is packed and they are ready to go. 'Oh yes, we intend to take the pram out often.' Mum proudly smiles down at her sleeping baby.

'I was thinking more about in a year's time. Whether we will see you walking with her or...' The end of the sentence remained unsaid, hanging in the air between them.

Mum says nothing. Her smile is gone. She doesn't manage to say another word. The joy of taking her new baby home and showing her off has evaporated and the strain of an uncertain future creeps over her again.

The midwife's comments make her insides shake as though someone has kicked her hard in the stomach. Why can't she just take her little daughter home like all the other new Mums and Dads?

Why can't she enjoy the unique smell of new-born baby, and look forward to people's comments about such a mop of dark hair and her beautiful delicate fingers? Why can't she enjoy the changes and development in her baby as the days pass, without being constantly reminded about something which is nothing more than speculation from a midwife who hasn't seen this sort of thing before and has no idea what the diagnosis might bring in the future?

Why can't Mum and Dad be given a farewell hug and reassuring words like *Go home and enjoy! It will be all right, you'll see! When the time comes we will help you through it!*

At home there is no professional to talk with the family, to ask how things are going, or tell them about particular things to be aware of. They return to normality as best they can and sometimes manage to forget about what lies around the corner.

Central Institute for Cerebral Palsy
13 September 1977

Dr Ole Haga
Nordfjord Hospital

Thank you for your letter regarding Turis Nygård's daughter and the X-rays which I return.

I have discussed the problem with Dr Hellum, who advises the difficult art of wait and see. This type of congenital scoliosis has a good prognosis and increase to the curvature is unusual. I advise that repeated X-rays in a year and annually if necessary should be adequate management of the condition. Treatment is not advised.

I am pleased to hear you like your job; I sometimes envy you the variety of cases you see.

Yours sincerely

Gunnar

Nordfjord Hospital
17 February 1978

Dr Hellum
Crown Princess Martha's Institute

Regarding Anne Pia Nygård, born 10 August 1977

Diagnosis: Congenital Scoliosis

Dear Colleague,

In September 1977 Gunnar Oftedal asked you to review a case and X-rays.

According to my information from Gunnar that this type of scoliosis is normally not progressive and we should take new X-rays in a year. We have done so and I include both the new and the original X-rays. There appears to have been a progression or it could be that she has learned to walk? That could perhaps give the impression of progression?

There is otherwise normal mental and motoric development. I am writing in collaboration with the parents, and have said to them that you may or may not need to see the patient in Oslo.

Many thanks for your help.

For information: the X-rays were taken lying down.

Yours sincerely

Ole Sverre Haga
Paediatrician

15 November 1978
Note to Dr Haga:

Outpatient visit regarding her scoliosis. Developmentally she is fine, more than adequate mentally, and seems like a pleasant child. Over cor there is an apparently phys. murmur grade 1-2 at the le. sternal border.

She has her scoliosis and a fairly deep Lumbar lordosis causing her abdomen to protrude. Short neck, head circumference 47.0cm equivalent to the 50th percentile, length 72 cm equivalent to the 2.5th percentile, weight 10kg equivalent to 50th-75th percentile.

X-rays taken of column. Previous pictures cannot be found in the card index at present; when they are found I will send them to Dr Hellum at Crown Princess Martha's Institute. He can decide whether to see the child.

Over cor there is an apparently phys. murmur grade 1-2 at the le. sternal border.

13 February 1979

Dr Hellum
Crown Princess Martha's Institute

Regarding Anne Pia Nygård born 10 August 1977

Dear Dr Hellum,

On 15 November 1978 I sent a letter enquiring whether you could assess the above patient who has a congenital scoliosis. Her parents have not heard from Crown Princess Martha's Institute and we wonder whether you have received the letter.

If you have received the letter and it will still be some time before you can assess the child, it would be good if you give us a hint regarding the approximate time scale.

Yours sincerely

Ole Sverre Haga
Paediatrician

Crown Princess Martha's Institute
9 July 1979

Copy: Dr I Bjerkreim
Sophies Minde

Paediatrician Ole Sverre Haga
Nordfjord Hospital

I have received a request to see Anne-Pia Nygård, born on 10 August 1977 with congenital scoliosis.

I do not remember replying to this request previously. Scoliosis is usually investigated and treated at Sophies Minde Orthopaedic Hospital. I will therefore forward your request to Dr Bjerkreim there.

Yours faithfully

Dr Cato Hellum
Junior Consultant

Nordfjord Hospital
8 August 1979

To the parents of Anne-Pia Nygård,

I hereby enclose a copy of correspondence regarding Anne-Pia.

Dr Hellum writes in his letter of 9 July 1979 that the papers have been sent to Dr Bjerkreim at Sophies Minde hospital.

If you do not hear anything from them by the beginning of September you or I ought to get in touch with them.

Yours sincerely

O.S. Haga
Central Institute for Cerebral Palsy

FIRST OPERATION

Norway has little experience of people with this diagnosis. Germany, on the other hand, has progressed further with treating curvature of the spine. When surgery was being considered it was natural for Dr Haga to investigate the possibility of carrying out the operation in Germany. The response from hospital doctors in Norway was negative. 'We can gain equally good results from such an operation here,' they said, 'there is no need to go to Germany.'

She needed to grow a bit more before such an operation could be carried out. Her back needs to be longer before they stiffen it. Up until then the scoliosis is to be treated with a corset.

But at the first outpatient appointment at Sophies Minde Orthopaedic Hospital they find a tight fibre by the coccyx on the X-rays they take. If the fibre is not cut now she will lose the feeling in her legs by the age of 12 or 13. They are allowed to celebrate Christmas at home but, when January arrives, her mother takes her back to Oslo where the necessary operation awaits. She is moved from Sophies Minde, the orthopaedic hospital, to Ullevaal Hospital, Oslo's main teaching hospital.

They wait for what seems like an eternity before the time comes for the operation. Mum goes with them as they roll the bed down the corridor, into the lift and down to the floor with the operation theatres. The bed has cot sides and in the bed a two-year-old dressed in a white hospital gown holds the bars. Her face shows no sign that she knows what is happening as she watches her Mum. Then the big double doors close behind the two-year-old's bed and the green-clad staff. Mum is not allowed in here.

Nervously and with a lump in her throat, Mum occupies herself by wandering around in the city. The capital city would normally be a rare luxury but not today. She barely notices the landmarks and the shops. She stops and looks at clothes but her mind is not on shopping. Her thoughts are somewhere else entirely, not here in the streets. Coming into town was meant to shorten the wait for her, to give her a distraction and allow her to believe, at least for a minute or two, that life is normal and that she is out shopping for pleasure. The distraction doesn't work.

After a couple of hours Mum goes back to the hospital. It feels like years since she left her two-year-old in the doctor's gloved hands. Her nerves eventually evaporate when they say the operation has gone well. Now her two-year-old has got to lie still on her tummy for seven days. Luckily she is not a very active child and so the days pass without incident. Dressed only in a jumper and tights she lies with her nappy-clad bottom sticking up in the air. Aunt Grete comes with toys and, through the bars, the two-year-old looks like a big doll in a heap of other toys.

A week later

Mum bends right down and stretches her arms out. Has her two-year-old forgotten how to walk? Her fears that disappeared a week ago are back, she sees the two-year-old take her first wobbly steps away from the doctor and towards her. Again her nerves melt away in the smile they all share as the child takes a couple of steps and falls into her Mum's arms.

A new weekend brings with it a welcome couple of days away from the hospital. Aunt Grete collects them in her car. Grete is married to Dad's older brother Harald. They have three children: Christine, Heidi and Linda. At home with Grete and Harald's family in Oslo, Mum and her two-year-old can relax. No need to think about needles and pain, all the waiting or what is going to happen next. Aunt Grete and Uncle Harald's house is full of animals. Budgies, dogs and rabbits. The perfect distraction.

FIRST CORSET

After the operation they moved her back to Sophies Minde hospital and it was there that they made her first tiny corset. The corset looked like a big belt with laces to hold it firmly in place and iron in the lining at the back. She was to have it on almost all the time. To start with it was for a few hours at a time so she could get used to it, adding more and more hours until it was on almost constantly.

She was the first-ever patient down in the orthopaedic ward to fall asleep while they were making the plaster mould! Lying on the treatment bench, she was rolled first in a gauze bandage dipped in warm, soft plaster. Gentle hands and a warm smile seem miles away from painful needles and doctors with cold stethoscopes.

Years later Dad finds a post card in the post when he is on his way home from work. It is addressed to 'Mr Atle Nygård and family'. On the front of the card was a picture of flowers and a bible verse. On the back was the neat and precise handwriting of an older person. The card was from Alf. He worked at Sophies Minde orthopaedic hospital and had been one of the people who made some of the corsets for the little girl from when she was two until she was ten.

Dear Family,
Thank you so much for the flowers and kind words,
As one of the 'ordinary' staff I was overwhelmed.
I have been unwell for the last three months so I have not been able to write until now.
I have started work again half-days and I hope to keep it up until the summer.
Say Hi to Pia for me!
Best wishes

FITS

During her first three years the little one has two severe epileptic fits for which nobody can find a cause. They come without warning. Her eyes roll backwards into her head, she froths at the mouth, and is unconscious for hours afterwards.

The first time she has a fit the doctors are out on strike. Mum and Dad do not have a telephone but fortunately Aunt Jorunn and Uncle Villie are visiting from Bergen. They manage to calm everyone down and head off to the doctor's surgery. When they get there they are told to go home again, as there is no doctor to see them. The best they can offer is a retired nurse who comes back home with them to be on the safe side.

Still unconscious the child is laid on the settee in the lounge. Nobody knows whether it is meningitis or if there will be permanent damage from being unconscious for so long. The only thing to do is to wait and see what happens when she wakes up. If she wakes up. And she does, suddenly and with a shake. Her body starts shaking, her eyes return to normal and begin to focus. Nobody knows what has happened or why but she seems OK, almost as if she has woken after a nap.

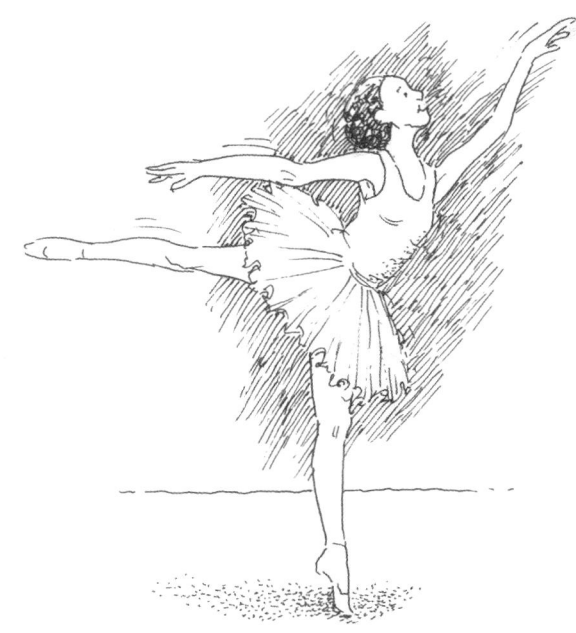

As she grows she is still small, and since there is very little room in her upper body she has a distended tummy and her spine shows itself as a hunch in her back.

She starts to compare her tummy with her big brother's and her little brother's tummies when they are in the bath together. She wonders why she is so much fatter than they are. Their tummies are flat like pancakes; they even go in a bit when they're sitting, make wrinkles. Her tummy sticks out all the time like a balloon, but she doesn't dare ask Mum why because she's afraid that her brothers will laugh at her. She doesn't want Mum to tell her she is fat. A ballerina can't be fat.

She sits so close to the TV that her nose almost touches it and watches the ballerinas gracefully jump from toe to toe into the strong arms of a man who is always there in the right place at the right time. Her secret dream is to be like that! 'This one will be a ballerina' say Mum and Dad as they wink at each other.

Though ballet is only on the TV, she does gymnastics in the gym hall. When she is here, she doesn't feel glamorous. She fumbles her way through the moves as best she can. The blue leotard feels good to have on and the small shows are a highlight as she shows Mum and her grandparents what she has learnt. If she could just manage to keep up.

One day a new family come to the gym training. They have two children, a boy, a girl and their parents. They are all true blonds, as if they each had a halo of shining white hair. They had warm smiles and were polite; she thinks they must be the perfect family. In that family everybody joins in together. Perfect children, perfect parents. Nobody is ever grumpy, no arguments, the perfect family. She can't take her eyes off them for the whole session.

Do I remember right?

It could be that she doesn't dare to look at them for the whole training session, afraid of not being worthy of them, as if Jesus comes with his family to see how normal people are getting on.

Every Friday there is a kids' club up at Bertel Farm. Alvhild and Oddrun make cocoa and squash for the twenty-odd children in the area who come charging in through the door, throwing off their outdoor clothes as they go. A heap of coats and a heap of boots and shoes left in the entrance is evidence of their arrival. Names noted down in a little book and in front of the name, a number. If you come through the door seventh you get a number seven in front of your name, if you are first you get a number one.

A letter has arrived and Alvhild reads it out. The letter is from a missionary in Africa who writes that we all must continue to do God's work; it is important to tell people about Jesus. That is what good Christians do.

Oddrun reads out in a sympathetic voice about people whose life is difficult but who love to dance and sing and thank God for the few things they have. They can teach us a lot about being thankful. What can we thank God for?

The first to arrive at the kids' club usually grab the places behind the sliding doors in the other lounge. There they sit half forgotten; they can wriggle and giggle before anyone says hush. They haven't heard the question.

After a bible story and something to eat, Alvhild goes around with a bowl with folded, numbered pieces of paper in it. The person who got the prize last time brings a little present to be the prize this time. Some sweets, a nice rubber or some chocolate. The children look at the prizes and dream that they will win that evening. Somebody draws a number and reads it out. There is a great sense of anticipation in the room as Alvhild checks in her little book to see who is lucky enough to have their name beside the number.

'*You* won what I brought. I really wanted to have it myself – you're so lucky!'

On the day of rest we have to get up early to go to Sunday school. There is more talk of Jesus and God and everything we have to do and everything we mustn't do to be good Christians. All this Christianity business is a bit difficult to understand. Not that it's difficult to understand the stories; they're stories and you have to believe stories. She doesn't question the virgin birth, or the Holy Spirit coming to the disciples, but she can't quite understand why Ragnhild says she doesn't believe in God. Doesn't everyone believe in Him? Does Ragnhild think that Alvhild and Oddrun, Bertel and Harald are lying, or talking about something they know nothing about?

Since she believes all the stories she has no reason to question whether you go to hell if you take God's name in vain. In the school playground, every time she hears someone say, 'O my God!' the words stick in her mind. Even though she has not said the words, they stay there and they grate just like when you can't stop thinking about all the things you don't want to think about. Pretending she has not heard doesn't help. Neither does it help to look busily at other people. She has to pray quickly that He won't be upset by the empty words that have been thoughtlessly used. It is a sin to take His name in vain.

Playtime might go something like this in her head:

(Someone shouts)	'Oh my God!'
(She silently prays)	'Lord God… thank you for today. Amen!
(Another says)	'Oh my God!'
(She silently prays)	'Lord God… look after my family and everyone in the world. Amen!'
(She hears)	'Oh my God!'
(She silently prays)	'Lord God… it is nice weather today… and… and… and we are having maths last lesson; let it be better than yesterday. Amen!'
(She hears someone say)	'Oh my God!'
(She needs to pray silently)	'Lord God … I am not sure what to say now, but thank you for everything you have created. Amen!'

S he sits on the swings with Ragnhild and they sing.

I was just eight when it happened
I heard an unforgettable song on the radio.
Everyone over thirty must remember singing this:

Oooo I love you baby, I love you so.
I need you honey, don't ever let me go!

My first English lesson from the radio was, 'Oooo I love you!'

Wooden walkie-talkies with a nail for an aerial and buttons painted on. These were used to spy on people going past on the street. Ragnhild and she warn each other about aliens who dare to land on planet earth and invade their territory. They also have a secret detective club which has an exclusive membership card with a space for their name and fingerprint. They make up the crimes they are to solve.

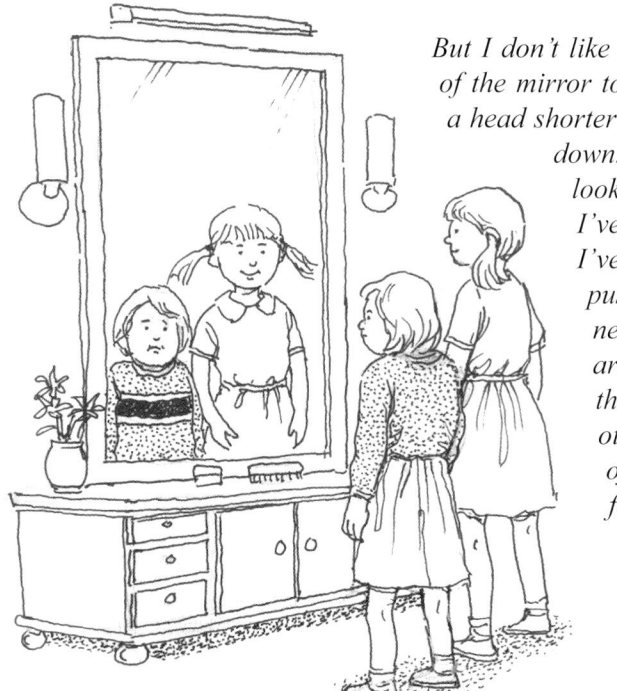

But I don't like it when we stand in front of the mirror to see who is tallest. I am a head shorter than her. I feel squashed down. Where is my neck? I look just like Barbie when I've pulled her head off; when I've put her head back on I've pushed it too far down her neck. The broken Barbies are still in the collection but they aren't as nice as the other ones. Here, in front of the mirror, I know how it feels to be Broken Barbie.

THE BEDROOM

At home there are the boys and her. Sometimes she has wished there was someone else to be on her side. She doesn't see the fun in war games with Lego, or making a fort to play Cowboys and Indians with plastic figures that never let go of their guns or spears. It always ends up with her getting bored of playing war games and wandering off. Then the boys get cross because she has gone before the war is over. Computer games are boring too when she has to watch the boys for such a long time before it is her turn.

It is better to be alone in her room. She can hide from everyone and everything. It is her world. She reads and disappears into the story to escape from her thoughts. In stories she can see things and experience things through others rather than be herself. She can widen her horizons and yet never go further than the sofa or the quilt on her bed.

One day the bed is changed for a sofa bed with a drawer under and a shelf above it. She turns some of the shelf into a Barbie room. *California Barbie* sits in her pink deck chair and enjoys the view of the room as she waits for her lover to come and leave again before Ken gets home from work. The rest of the Barbies are lined up on the floor ready to make their entrance. She sits cross-legged on the floor, and every doll is involved in intricate plots where love and jealousy provide the backdrop and there is the occasional murder. In the background the cassette player creates the atmosphere. Sometimes it could be Dad's film music with songs from the '50s and '60s; at other times Swedish pop hits: *Dear Dad, don't drink any more, I can't watch Mum cry again... I had a girl, Donna was her name, since she's been gone I've never been the same, 'cause I love my girl – Oh Donna where can you be?*

She likes to play alone best, so that she can let her imagination run free. And anyway there aren't many in the neighbourhood who play much with Barbies. Out of the local children she is usually with Ragnhild. The rest are mostly boys like her brothers; two from next door and some from the other houses down the street. She isn't always allowed to be with them either. She doesn't really like war games, where you have to run and hide, very much at all. When she is playing outside she is easily tired and she has trouble keeping up. Sometimes she suddenly needs to wee, but because she doesn't want to spoil the game by going home she tries to hang on until the last moment. She has also got a bigger and stiffer corset now; it makes her feel like a robot. She overheats in it and it makes her itch so she sticks a knitting needle down her back to scratch with.

The wardrobe has something in it that no one else knows about. At the back, behind her dresses, there is a secret door that only *she* knows about. Nobody else can see it. When Mum puts her clothes away, she sits on the floor and thinks that Mum can't see what is right in front of her nose. The secret room behind the dresses is a good place to be. There she can play with special friends without getting tired or needing to wee. They are always in a good mood, they don't tell her off, and when she is with them she is in charge.

She always locks her bedroom door, afraid that someone will burst in and disturb her and wonder what she's up to with her nose in the wardrobe. Anyway her family really do need to learn to knock.

She loves to be alone in her room. It is different being there alone, better than anywhere else. She can be alone and yet with others here. Out there she can feel alone even when she is with other people.

Imaginary monsters fight against good. It is OK to watch them in a film, but I know that if I should get into a situation like that I would be petrified and run off. At times like that I would never manage to be a hero. Just the thought of it makes me feel sick as I lie hidden under my duvet. There is a tiny crack, just big enough to let in enough air to breathe. She knows the dark ones are standing around the bed. They whisper in her head. 'Mum, do you sometimes hear voices in your head?'

I could never be brave. I am too cowardly and too scared for that. In the final battle between good and evil I lie under the duvet and hardly dare breathe.

Sometimes I imagine there is a boy sleeping, dreaming my life. He is a giant and I am so little that there is room for me in his dreams. I can visualise him as he lies asleep in bed, on his side with his face towards the room. His gentle breathing makes the duvet go up and down in an even rhythm. Blue-and-white-striped pyjamas. Short blonde hair with a fringe that's sticking up and over to one side. He has the same stupid whirl of hair at the front that I have.

I can't see his family near him. Just the boy sleeping in his bed, dreaming of me. Of course it isn't important, but I bet he has loads of friends to play with when he is awake. He is probably really popular and he's dreaming about me! The most important thing is that he keeps me alive. He is real and I am a dream. It's easier that way. All the stupid things will be gone when he wakes up, they won't matter any more. It is important that the real one of us is the popular one.

But he will soon wake and I will be gone.

I am not even afraid to think about that.

DINNER

Nothing must be missing at a meal time. Like when she comes home from school and the others have eaten all the sauce. She is furious and starts to cry. You just can't have fish fingers without sauce. Everything to do with food has to be just so and she has to have two helpings of dinner to have enough. Even though she gets a bit of a conscience when Mum drops broad hints that she's had enough, she still always has two helpings!

Today she has a friend round who also likes to play with Barbies. It isn't quite the same playing *Barbie* with someone else, but her guest wants to do that and she knows that when the girl has gone she will have the dolls to herself again, it is therefore OK to share. Anyway, she always gives in, never dares to stop other people having their own way. She only ever argues with her family. Besides, she likes having friends over.

Her visitor goes home at dinner time but wants someone to go part of the way with her. Of course one doesn't refuse to do that, even though it is dinner time right now. Before they go she pops into the kitchen to see what is for dinner. Mum is at work so Dad is making dinner. Chips!

She asks them to make sure they save enough for when she gets back. But by the time she gets back, not more than fifteen minutes later, everything has been gobbled up! She is angry and upset. It feels like somebody has hit her in the head. Like the most important thing she owns has been stolen. She vents her frustration hysterically. How dare they! What can comfort her now? What is there to look forward to for the rest of the day?

'You would never manage as a cook in Africa, you would eat all the food yourself!' says Dad. But they don't feel the unease in her body when she doesn't have that second helping.

'Get something else then!' It's easy for them. They don't understand why she is so cross. They were hungry and she wasn't even there!

She sits on the grass, watching the other children playing a football match. Should she go over to Dad at half time and ask for an ice cream? She can hear his voice thundering out of the loud speaker. Someone has scored. People clap. The sun warms. The corset is so itchy.

'Why do your shoulders go right up to your ears?' A boy materialises in front of her. She knows who he is. One of those who dares to say anything. One of those who's not afraid of anyone or anything. She can't say a word. She has never really thought about why her shoulders come right up to her ears. They're just like that. It is just that she has a bend in her spine that nobody else has and now she has a bigger and stiffer corset that makes her feel and move like a robot. It is so big that she needs help to scratch her back, even with a knitting needle. It is just the way it is.

Now she is embarrassed. Why is it people always have to notice her shoulders? She is so much more than just that. For example, she could read and write before she went to school. In year one there were only two children who could do that - her and one other. They got an extra exercise book with more difficult writing exercises in it. She liked that book.

At home she, just like her mother and grandmother, reads the short stories and true stories in magazines. She loves the short stories which often include young, beautiful girls and gorgeous men who always end up together. And she likes the true stories that seem to be so tragic that they also are good. She can imagine just how she will be and how she will behave when she grows up. Far in the future, aged seventeen or maybe eighteen with jeans, a jumper and a short jacket over the top. She will spike her fringe up and she will buy curling tongs or have a perm at the hairdressers. She will wear huge earrings and lots of eye makeup and thick rouge on her cheeks. Of course she will be cute and clever and have a queue of drooling boys after her. Just like in the magazine stories. But she only has eyes for George Michael and he only has eyes for her. The boys will stare at her because she is beautiful and not because she has shoulders right up to her ears.

Mum took the boys and me to the park.

'IS IT TRUE THAT YOU'RE IN LOVE WITH ME, ANNE-PIA?'

The boy was standing at the top of the slide and was shouting down. They hadn't even got in through the gate. As the tiny park resounded with his words, it seemed all the children in the park stopped what they were doing and looked. It couldn't have been many seconds before I reacted but it felt like time had stood still. Everyone was looking at me. I looked angrily at Paul who was mindlessly picking at his shoulder. He hadn't said anything!

'No!' I automatically screamed back at the boy. I didn't dare look towards where he was standing in case he said something else. Without meeting all those eyes staring in my direction, I quickly went in through the gate and over the playground to the building where rucksacks hang. I wished, as I walked, that I could stay in all day today so I wouldn't have to face the others. Wouldn't have to meet their teasing stares.

When I came back out everyone was busy playing again. What was that feeling I had, relief or disappointment?

Dad can sing and play the guitar. In his youth he was in a band that played concerts and went on tour.

She sits on the corner of the settee and he gets out his guitar. They have their repertoire ready.

Dad, what if the sun goes out, what would happen then?

If the sun goes out there will be crying everywhere, everything will suddenly be dark and cold. But if the wind lifted up every tear that fell, the sun would start to shine again.

But Dad, what if there was no wind, what will happen then?

If there was no wind then the clouds in the sky would stop. No yachts would sail, no kites would fly. But the grass would reach high up and then the wind would soon blow again.

But Dad, what if the grass withers, what would happen then?

If the grass withers, the earth would indeed be a sad place. What, after all, is a place where nothing grows? But our God is good and his love is great, just see, the grass would grow again.

But Dad, what if there was no love, what would happen then?

If there was no love the wind would not blow, the grass wouldn't grow and the sun wouldn't shine. That is why you and I must always love each other. The world needs love today, hmmm, the world needs love today, hmmm, the world needs love today, hmmm.

Dad says 'Helge Nilsen sings that song with his son. He is the one who sings with Rune Larsen, you know.'
'Can we sing that song too,' she asks.

In a room in the hospital, where the white beds are,
Lies a weak little girl, gentle and kind with golden hair.

She's won all their hearts as she lies there so gentle and kind,
In her pain she does not complain, a brave and holy child.

And she whispers to her doctor as he stands beside her bed,
'Will I be home for Easter, will I be well by then?'

The doctor answers, 'no, my child, I don't think so
Perhaps by Pentecost you will be home with Mum.'

Pentecost comes with its green trees, fields and meadows full of wild flowers
But she lies there still, a prisoner in her hospital bed.

And when the autumn shakes her fragile frame
She sometimes asks if autumn could be her time for home.

The doctor's only answer is to stroke her golden hair
He barely hides his tear-filled eyes as he turns away and goes.

As the bells toll Christmas in, peace on earth can now begin,
The white bed lies empty; her voice will be for ever still

Now she rests in her grave beneath a snowy blanket,
Now the wait is at last over, she is safe at home with God.

SUMMER HOLIDAYS

Every summer the family go to Askøy Island to visit Uncle Leif, Aunt Kari, Jan and Anne. They also spend a couple of days on Sotra with Grandma who lives upstairs from Uncle Villie and Aunt Jorunn. Grandma, Dad's Mum, uses strange words or gives words slightly different meanings. She is going to spend a penny when she means she is going to the toilet and she has to 'remember to take all her pills'.

Grandma always calls her Anne-Pi. It is as though Grandma hasn't the energy to put the end on her name, although it is only one extra letter. She is never quite sure because Grandma can be a tease.

Her cousins on Sotra are so much older than her that they don't really play together. Visiting Grandma is the reason for going there. But on Askøy Island her cousins are about the same age so they play together all day.

Anne has a big drawer full of comics. There are so many that it is impossible to read your way through the heap. One evening, as they lie reading before they go to sleep, Anne says that the one who wakes up first tomorrow has to wake the other one straight away. She agrees, and means it. The problem is that she wakes first the next morning and when she looks across at her sleeping cousin she doesn't dare wake her. What if Anne is cross at being woken so early? Some people are grumpy before they are properly awake in the morning and regret asking anyone to wake them. She doesn't think Anne will be grumpy – she is never grumpy with her. Just to be on the safe side, in case it is too early, she lies down again and stays still until she hears Anne begin to wriggle and stretch. She can pretend they wake at the same time. That's a much better plan.

At the edge of her aunt and uncle's garden there are wild blueberries. They have just got the latest copy of *Barbie Magazine*, which has two pages in it on the language of flowers. Blueberries are not flowers, but they can eat the berries as they lie in the grass and read about flowers. Red roses – I love you, yellow roses – I don't love you, forget-me-nots – friendship, lily of the valley – I have a secret, pink carnations – I am thinking of you.

They read the names and meanings to each other and pretend to give flowers. She brings the game alive and Anne laughs at her antics. 'Mum you have to see Anne-Pia's funny faces!' shouts Anne and drags her in to where Auntie is ironing. 'Show Mum your faces!' encourages Anne, laughing and, despite a sudden wave of shyness, she tries her best to recreate the funny faces she made in the garden. She is relieved when Auntie also thinks it is funny.

Dad goes with her to the outpatient appointments in Oslo. They go at least a couple of times each year.

It is not very long since their local airport opened, though it was before she was born. The airport is so little that it can only take small planes like the Twin Otter which they call *Seagull* and the Dash 7. But it's plenty big enough for planes to Oslo. The world was smaller back then. It is special to be going on an aeroplane. Not many of her friends have ever flown, so she feels special when she has to fly to Oslo at least twice a year. It is a big event to go to Oslo, the big capital city. She hasn't ever seen other children from the area on board.

The taxi is ordered. It is really early. The rest of the family are still asleep. Mum comes sleepily down in her dressing gown to say good bye before they leave. At the airport, *Seagull* has been waiting for hours but is now ready for a new trip.

The feeling of flying is as exciting every time when you are small. There is a kind of fear as she walks across the runway to the fuselage that will lift them thousands of feet into the air. The adults have to bend to get in but she can walk unhindered through the doorway. The adults have to stoop as they make their way to the nearest seat, fasten their seatbelts and check that the sick bag is handy. Then they smile and nod to the other passengers around them. 'So you are off on a trip today?' 'Yes, I think it will be good flying weather.' 'Yes we're off to Oslo again.' As they wipe their sweaty palms on their trousers and fiddle with their clothes.

She sits next to Dad. Big safe Dad; she snuggles up to him and falls asleep once the initial excitement of taking off is over. Before the plane moves she is sitting nicely and waiting, muscles tense. Her whole body vibrates as the motor revs up. The propellers spin faster and faster and then the plane begins to move. They taxi to the end of the runway, the plane turns in a wide arc, then stops. The engine thunders, the propellers have become invisible. They are pressed back into their seats as the plane shoots forward so fast that the plane lifts from the runway! Dad has given her some gum to chew so her ears don't pop. If they come into bad weather then the sick bags will be needed. The trip takes a couple of hours and includes a stop-over at Sogndal or Ørsta where they change to a bigger plane. On the big plane she is given a jigsaw and a badge, as well as a carton of orange juice.

Once they have landed Dad fusses his way to the taxi queue. Once in the back seat he says 'Sophies Minde Hospital' to the driver and the car moves off, the airport soon behind them. The radio is on in the background. A friendly voice with a southern accent gives the weather report and traffic news. Messages flow in to a little machine that ticks along. From her seat she tries to peep at the messages without dad or the driver noticing. There is heavy traffic and several people wanting taxis to the airport. It is easiest to read it unnoticed when they have a driver who likes to chat. Then she can listen to the radio and read the messages while the adults talk. It is mostly the driver who chats, asks questions and talks about things she thinks are boring. Dad doesn't like the driver chatting – he nods, smiles and gives short answers. She can tell from his voice that he would rather disappear into his own thoughts as he sits there on the back seat.

Then she thinks about their journey home after their last trip to Oslo. At the airport they had been stopped at security and taken to one side. 'What have you got there young lady?' asked one of the customs officers suspiciously as he pressed her tummy. They could all hear the hard sound. The customs officers raised their eyebrows to Dad. He realised straight away what they thought. They thought he was using his daughter to smuggle something. To prove their innocence he lifted her jumper so they could see the corset. He explained to them what it was and why she has to wear it. They were hastily allowed to go, with a glance that had suddenly changed to compassion.

OUTPATIENT AT SOPHIES MINDE
ORTHOPAEDIC HOSPITAL

Butterflies start to fly around in her tummy as they get nearer to the hospital. The familiar building comes in to view. Dad asks for a receipt and pays the driver. He always give the driver more than the cost of the journey, even when the driver has talked all the way. The driver thanks them, slams closed the car doors and hurries back to the airport.

I'm sure it's true that Dad is fed up with always having to wait around at Sophies Minde. First they go to the window and announce their arrival, where they are told to take a seat and wait to be called into the X-ray department. After what seems like ages her name is called out and they are shown behind big doors. Then they have to wait again until a lady comes and shows them to the room with the X-ray machine. 'Back for more pictures, are you?' smiles the X-ray lady as she presses a small cold and heavy plate to the girl's tummy with white tape. Her naked back is pressed against another cold plate. The X-ray machine is positioned above her body and adjusted to the right height and distance. 'Stay still and hold your breath until I tell you!' The X-ray lady puts a big, heavy apron on Dad then they both go behind a door and look at her through a window. Soon they come out again and the X-ray lady takes the plate from her back and pulls out another plate from it. That is the picture which is to be developed. They repeat the whole thing a couple more times in different positions. She has to stand with both her hips in to the cold plate and her tummy pressed against it. She is cold as she waits for the pictures to be developed. Waits until the people who look at the pictures are satisfied; only then she is allowed to put her trousers and jumper on and leave the room.

Once the X-rays are done they have to wait in Dr Lange's waiting room. This one is the longest wait. There is always a long queue of people in the waiting room. Sometimes people who arrive after her are called in before her. She is always the last name to be called. Dad asks Dr Lange if it is possible for them to come in sooner, since they have had such a long journey and have to make the plane home. 'We save the best 'til last,' is always the same answer.

Dr Lange is an elderly man with grey hair. He has an accent from eastern Norway and a calm deep voice. She likes him because he is always pleased to see her and he makes her feel like a very special patient. There is another doctor in the office. A short, chubby man who sits on a stool and leans on his stick. He is the exact opposite of Dr Lange; one long, one short, one round and one thin. Once she has taken her jumper and corset off she is sent back and forth between these two doctors. They feel and squeeze her back. The X-rays that were taken earlier hang on the illuminated board and show just how crooked her spine is.

The pattern on the curtains is of flowers in two or three different colours. Red, of course, brown, green and a pale background. They hang heavy. She stares at the curtains while the doctors talk. Whenever she hears something her Dad and Mum are discussing quietly in the next room, Dad says that she leaves her ears on the table. Her ears are now on the doctor's big table, but her thoughts are somewhere else entirely. Perhaps at home. Not 210 home or in bed at 210, her room in the hospital. Maybe she is at home with her sister and brothers – or maybe she is at 'home' with Linda, Heidi and Christine, her aunt, uncle and all the animals. She is lucky to have two families. Two homes. There is however a third home; Sophies Minde where she has her own room and people who look after her. But here she is alone in a different way to when she is at home with all her things around her. Nine others share room 210. Nine others to be alone with. She thinks about different things here than when she is in her room at home. At Sophies Minde she thinks about home. At home she thinks about imaginary things.

The doctor moves across to her, rolls easily on his stool. He has to stand up to feel her back. He squeezes her tummy and back then asks something about the corset. She smiles and replies. She looks at Sister Kari who smiles back. Lifts up her arms one after the other, turns round slowly, then she is to sit down so the doctor can check her reflexes. She looks across to Sister Kari who also has sat down. Smiles trustingly at her. The doctor asks more questions and she answers as best she can. Hopes she gives the right answer. Sister Kari says something. The doctor and the Sister talk and she can get dressed. 'Can I ring home this evening?' she wonders as she looks at the grey telephone on the desk. 'We have exactly the same type of telephone at home,' she thinks, 'except it's black.' She imagines Mum dialling the number to Sophies Minde. Round and round until all the numbers are dialled. 'Mum will ring soon,' she thinks, and almost expects the patients' telephone behind the door to begin to ring immediately. She is impatient to be finished so she can wait in the hall for the phone to ring and the voice to ask to speak to her.

She hasn't always got coins. Sometimes she puts in all the numbers one after another without putting the coins in first, just because she has nothing else to do. On one occasion there is a voice on the other end. She hadn't expected that. She is scared and hangs up. Scared that she might have rung abroad.

Sometimes she is allowed to ring home from the grey phone on the doctor's desk. Sister Kari dials 0 to the switchboard so they can give her a line out. Then she tells someone at the other end the number to Mum and Dad's phone. After a moment it rings both on the doctor's telephone and at home. Then Sister Kari gives her the receiver so she can wait until someone at home answers the rings with 'Nygård?'

Mostly she goes around the ward listening for the patients' phone to ring, then wondering if it will be trundled in to room 210 and across to her bed. But there are nine others in the room each waiting for the phone to ring. Nine others who have more people who want to ring them. She feels that most of the calls are to others, not to her.

'Sophies' has four floors

On the ground floor is the reception desk, check-in, outpatients, X-ray, doctors' surgeries, orthopaedic department and various waiting rooms.

She is on the first floor. As well as the children's ward there is the staff canteen. When Mum and Dad were here for assessments with her when she was younger, they weren't given refreshments, even though they might have to wait all day. It was only years later that parents with food slips were able to get themselves something to eat in the canteen. Physiotherapy is also on this floor.

In the hallways, as I was practicing my walking, I heard children's story cassettes. In this department I have almost nodded off as I lie on my tummy, peeping through a hole in the bench while my legs are bent and stretched.

On the second floor are the adult wards and the post-operative room.

In the adult ward everything is different. The smell. The people. The rooms. I don't like going up there.

Most of the third floor is empty. There is a classroom up here for school-age patients who are long-term inpatients. She has been here sometimes. Made plans for school work.

In the children's ward there are four big rooms. Room 207 has all the tiny babies who lie in their cots with their legs in traction; their parents sit by their cots and play with them, or try to talk comfortingly with them, so they might forget what is happening with their legs.

In room 208 is for children who are no longer toddlers but are not yet teenagers either. There are some in here too who are in traction. Others use a corset. Room 209 is the boys' room.

I am scared to walk past the boys' room, so I always hurry past it. I don't know how Hanne dares to stand in the doorway and look at the boys or talk to them. But I always stand beside Hanne. A little bit behind and to one side of her so the boys don't notice me. I like it when Hanne comes to work with her Mum. Inger Johanne is a real favourite because she is one of the nurses who 'care'. Inger Johanne works in 'my' room.

Room 210. This is the teenage girls' room. She is sometimes in room 208 and sometimes in 210, depending on friends, but 210 has become her regular room. She thinks it's kind of fun that she has been put in with teenagers when it will be a long time until she is a teenager. There is a TV above the door in all the rooms. In room 210 it is tuned to MTV and provides 'general entertainment' all day.

The older girls and boys who are there to have their legs lengthened have a long thing attached to their legs which they screw a little bit each day until their legs are as long as they need to be and they can take it off. Most of the girls in room 210 use a corset. Other children and teenagers have short arms or are missing a foot.

The nurses who work on this ward are always responsible for the same room. The ones in room 210 often make an extra-nice supper. Sometimes she is allowed to use the tea kitchen to make a meal with one of the nurses. Chocolate balls with oats. Then she is allowed to have apple juice from the fridge. She doesn't get apple juice at home.

On the long wall opposite are the toilets. Whenever she sits on the toilet she stares at the paper bags hanging beside the toilet roll. They have instructions in Norwegian, English and another language she doesn't recognise. She has no idea what the bags are for. The only thing she understands about them is that they must not be thrown down the toilet because they will block the toilet. So as not to do anything wrong she doesn't touch them. She sits on the toilet seat and wonders what you might put in one of these bags and then throw down the toilet.

THE BIG OPERATION

She is seven and it has been decided that they will carry out an operation to even out the scoliosis. Before setting off for Oslo she went to the hairdresser's and had her lovely long hair cut short. It had almost reached her bottom but it is short now. 'It will be more practical when you are going to be such a long time in hospital, have an operation and be in bed a lot.'

She is going to have a cage with a steel ring around her head and a steel ring round her middle. It is attached to her body with rods and with screws into her head.

They tell her about three other children who have had this operation. They tell her it is no problem to move even when the cage is round her. The boys who have had this operation were just as active, running and chasing with it on as though it wasn't there at all. She gets to meet a teenage girl who has now had the cage removed. The only hints that she has had the cage in the past are small scars.

On the evening before the operation she has a bath. In the middle of the floor in the communal bathroom for that ward is the bath tub. There is no lock on the door. A notice says vacant or engaged.

The next morning she has been fasting since midnight and, although she is too nervous to eat, it would have been nice to have some bread and a glass of chocolate milkshake for breakfast. It might be a long time until the operating theatre contacts the ward to say they are ready for her. She is already looking forward to the operation being over and being able to eat again. 'As soon as you wake up and come back to the ward again you can have something to eat,' the nurse replies when she asks. 'Is there anything special you'd like to eat when you are back again?'

She thinks about it.

The operation is a success. Two Harrington staves will be surgically put in at a later date. They will be attached to her spine to hold it firm. Dad is with her when she wakes from the anaesthetic but he has to fly back to Sandane that same evening.

It hurts when he goes. She is still sleepy and not properly awake after the anaesthetic but she knows that it is painful to think that Dad has to go. Then she sees him beside her bed again. She is so glad when he comes back that she thinks she is seeing things. Then she notices a strange man behind him. Dad says he met a journalist in the hallway who had stopped him. The journalist had heard about the special operation and wanted to take some pictures. Glad to have Dad back for a little while longer she allows the man to take pictures.

Some days later, back on the children's ward, four adjustable rods are screwed to the steel rings. This makes a cage. She can no longer move her head without her upper body moving too. She has become a human robot. For many months Dr Bjerkreim adjusts the rods on the cage. A few millimetres each day so that her spine slowly straightens up and the hump can disappear.

It doesn't take long to catch the media's attention. A journalist and a photographer come from a national newspaper to write a story about her. They bring a teddy and a little doll for her. They take pictures in the play room, in the doctors' consulting room, with Nurse Kari and Dr Bjerkreim, of her sitting smiling in front of an X-ray picture of her spine. The journalists ask all sorts of questions and she hopes she answers them properly.

Everyone on the children's ward waits with anticipation for the article to be published. She is in the play room when he rolls in, one foot resting on a cushion and sticking straight out. He tries to manoeuvre his wheelchair with only one hand, while with his other hand he is waving the newspaper. 'It's here,' he shouts. 'You're on the front page and there is even a colour photo!'

One day a Norwegian magazine comes to takes pictures of her and to write about her. That is the day that Grandma, Aunt Grete and Linda are visiting. It is a Friday and, as usual, she is going to stay with her aunt, uncle and cousins for the weekend. The journalists ask if they too can come along. Before long they are in the car and the journalists are following in the car behind, just like spies.

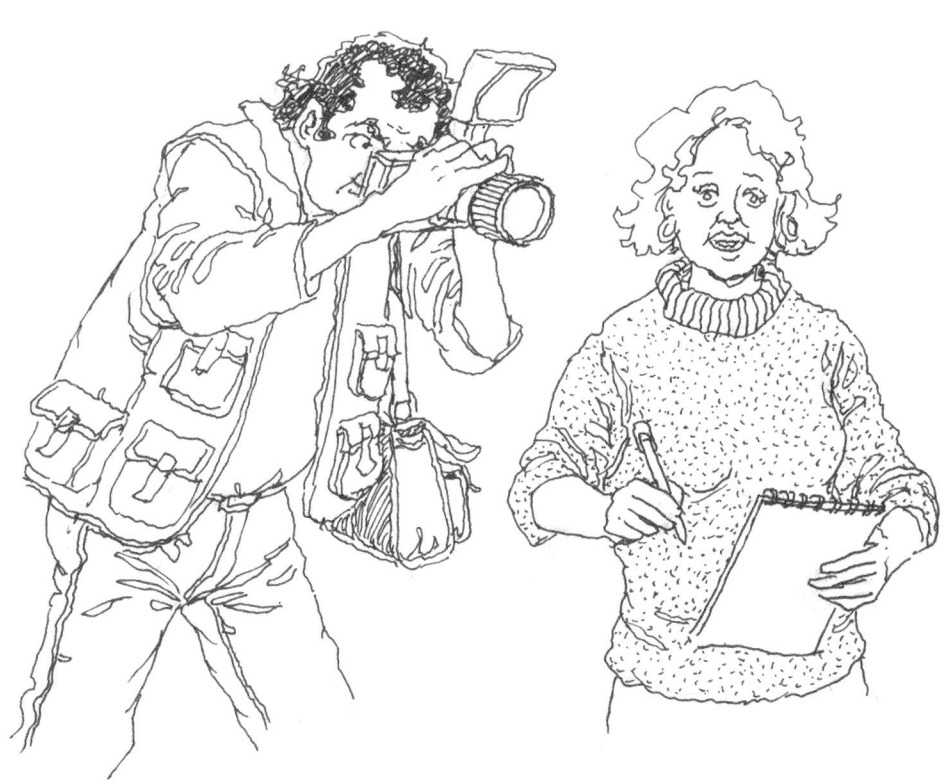

Special cage for 6-year-old: STRETCHED ANNE-PIA 8cm

'That's wrong, I'm seven!'

Anne-Pia must stay in her 'cage' until the summer. The doctors use the cage to straighten a large curve in her spine. Every day the seven-year-old is screwed one millimetre taller. To date she is eight centimetres taller. The cage is made up of four steel screws attached to her skull and two steel rods through her hips.

(...) With four solid steel screws fastened to her skull and two steel rods through her hips Anne-Pia draws attention at Sophies Minde hospital in Oslo.

'People ask if it hurts, but injections and operations are much worse,' says the young Miss Nygård.

It is true. Every time the needle lady comes to take a blood sample she has to have someone who will hold her other hand. Someone she can hold on tight to and pass the pain on to, someone who talks to her when she closes her eyes and turns away. She refuses to look until they say they are finished. Sometimes they don't say anything, and when she asks whether they are going to put the needle in soon, the nurse says they are finished.

In only a few months Anne-Pia has become 80mm taller. She will be a bit taller still but the doctors are almost finished with her treatment.

Rare
'Within two years she ought to be able to live a normal life. Gymnastics and sports should not be impossible,' says consultant Dr Bjerkreim.

'Anne-Pia's handicap is very rare. We see one such case every couple of years while five or six patients are treated with a halo-pelvic-head-hip stretch each year. We usually wait until the patient is 8-10 years old. Anne-Pia is the

youngest we have treated in this way at Sophies Minde,' explains ward sister Kari Hellum.

Patient

It was on 8 January that Anne-Pia came to Sophies Minde from Sandane in the county of Sogn & Fjordane. Living for six months in a hospital many miles from home can be a test of patience for children or adults but the seven-year-old passed with flying colours:

'I miss my sister Guro most of all. She is a baby, only eight months old,' she says.

'Of course I miss Mum and Dad too but it helps a bit because they at least come to visit. My aunt and uncle don't live too far from here and it is lovely when they come.'

Anne-Pia remembers the time when she was going to give little Guro a hug when she arrived with their parents for a visit. She was so pleased she forgot about the screws sticking out of her head. Fortunately Guro wasn't hurt.

'In five weeks I am having the cage removed and getting a corset. I will be able to go home before the summer.' She rushes on: 'In the autumn I am going to start in year two at school with Ragnhild and all my other friends.'

Anne-Pia has had a letter and lots of pictures from her classmates. She has stuck them on the wall with pictures from the other patients. They are of 'Anne-Pia with deluxe cage.'

When Anne-Pia arrived at Sophies Minde Hospital she had a curvature of the spine at her shoulder blades of almost 90 degrees. Now, after nearly three months treatment, her spine has only a 30-degree curvature. That is how it should be.

Two weeks ago Anne-Pia was operated on again, this time at Ullevaal Hospital in Oslo, where they have all the necessary equipment for big operations. They put in two rods called Harrington Staves. These tighten up her back and will prevent her from growing any more just there. These treatments have come from the USA and Hong Kong.

The results are extremely good. Even though it's unpleasant to go around with the cage for a few months, the other option would be to live with a significant curvature of the spine with little chance of living a 'normal' life.

IT IS MORE DIFFICULT AT NIGHT

Some of the night nurses have a reputation for being grumpy. These ones are not liked. One night when she is in pain after an operation the night nurse refuses to give her more pain killers. 'It is not long since you had some,' is all the nurse says before returning to her cigarettes in the staff room. No words of comfort, not even a smile. The girls in the room stare after her, angry and frustrated. It was they who called for help after hearing her crying quietly because of the pain. She would never have dared to say anything. She just tried to be quiet.

Because of the cage she lies on a mattress with grooves in. This means that when she lies down she is stuck and has to have help to turn over. In the night someone usually comes to move her sleepy body so she does not lie for too long in the same position. It starts to prickle somewhere on her body. She is uneasy and needs to move.

She often wakes feeling like that. She pulls the cord by her bed after thinking about whether to or not for a while. She hopes she doesn't disturb the night nurses while they are having their coffee or have just lit a cigarette, because they have just got chance to sit down and have a break.

If she pulls the cord just as the warm coffee is on its way down and the cigarette smoke on its way up, she can almost hear them through the walls, 'not again! There's no peace!' She can hear it in their footsteps as they approach room 210. She regrets pulling the bell cord the moment she has done it. Regrets disturbing them. The door to her room opens and lets in a strip of light. A hand gropes in the dark and turns the bell off, turns the lamp on which casts a grey light in the room, and looks to see who is awake. She lifts a hand to signal it is her that needs help.

'There needs to be two of us,' she says when I have explained in quiet whispers that I want to lie on my side. She disappears off to get the other night nurse. I lie there and study the 'Drama' posters as I pick out a bit of the picture in the light of my bedside lamp. Part of the picture remains only an outline. I have only heard a couple of this boy band's songs. The girl who had this bed before me must have left the poster behind. I like having something to look at.

I hope my light doesn't wake the others. Luckily I'm in a corner bed so I only have someone on one side of me. The others are further away and I hope they won't be too disturbed by the lamp. On the other hand, we are all used to being disturbed during the night.

When the night nurses return they stand one on either side of the bed. They each take an arm and pull her up into a sitting position so that the rods come out of the grooves in the bed. They put her legs over the edge of the bed and her bottom in the middle of the mattress. They help her to lie on the bed again, on her side this time and they ensure the rods are properly in the grooves. If they miss the grooves she has to sit up move a bit then they try again. They pull the cover over her, turn off the lamp and say goodnight.

The arm she is lying on starts to throb. She tries to sleep but soon realises that she won't be able to get off to sleep in that position. She tries to hang on a bit. She can't ring again as soon as the nurses have gone!

She tries to think about something else. Count sheep, anything. She has her back to the poster. The others are sleeping peacefully around her. No, she has to pull the bell again. Hopes they haven't just sat down. She can hear the bell from another room so they haven't stopped yet. It takes a while from when she pulls the cord until the nurses come. 'I want to lie on my back again.' The same procedure as last time. 'Try to sleep now,' the night nurse says, then she turns off the lamp and disappears. 'That's easy for her to say!'

The nights are long. She doesn't know how long it is before she sleeps but it doesn't seem to be long before she is woken by the day staff.

Suddenly the night was too short after all.

They are woken early, before the doctor's rounds. Up, washed, breakfast (bread and chocolate milkshake), watch TV, sometimes a blood test, wander around a bit. Watch some more TV, up and down in the lift, getting off on every floor. Look at the pictures – birds shaped from buttons, and the photographs of the staff hanging on the notice board – run fingers along the wall. Go into the play room, paint a plaster-of-Paris figure, do a picture. Back to the ward, watch MTV, have a drink, wait for dinner. Eat dinner. Want seconds. *Would like to go out.*

Goes to and fro in front of the staff office until someone notices her. *She would never ever dare to go in without permission.* Goes past, circles around it until someone notices and says: 'Come in Anne-Pia!' The best thing about being here is the nurses. They look after her, entertain her, talk to her. She sits in the office with them. They light a cigarette, two cigarettes, three cigarettes. Put hand cream on their hands.

They laugh together about something one of them says. The nurses are always in a good mood. They help her to forget herself, her loneliness, her home, for a while. The bell goes in one of the wards, someone knocks on the door. They see her sitting there, see that she is allowed to be with the nurses. She has to leave when it is time for a meeting, wander about a bit, run fingers along the wall, look at the pictures. She has other friends but none of them are here as long as she is.

Cathrine is often here. Her bones break easily, even when someone is a bit rough with her. Osteoporosis. That is why she is on the children's ward so much. People who don't know Cathrine think that she is three years old, even though she is actually two years older than Anne-Pia. When she isn't sitting in her bed, or being pushed around by her Mum, she uses her electric wheelchair. The two girls explore the hospital together and sometimes with others too. She often wanders around alone. It is Cathrine she thinks about when Dad and she sing the *Hospital Song* at home. The song has a sad ending, but even so she can't help but think about Cathrine and Sophies Minde Hospital.

WANDERING

She's been allowed around the back of the reception desk to see what it is like on the other side. When they get busy and she has to go again she stands outside and watches all the people and the taxis arriving. When she heads back up to the children's ward for dinner she sometimes meets the postman in the lift. The postman has a trolley full of post to be sorted. He gets out of the lift before her even though she is only going from the ground floor to the first floor. He presses a button that stops the lift between the two floors. He goes out of a door in the opposite wall to the one everyone else uses.

She tries to imagine what the post room is like. A secret room with lots of people sorting letters and parcels as they come along the conveyor belt. She thinks the children's ward gets the most parcels. Big and little 'thoughts' from people at home. *Get well soon! We are looking forward to you coming home! Buy yourself something nice with this money!* Letters from grandparents and classmates. 'A bit like Santa's grotto,' she thinks.

The daily wandering around the different floors is because the days are long. She needs to find something to do. During the day, the ground floor is always full of people. Three of them from the children's ward take a wheelchair each from the hallway. These big hospital wheelchairs have always got something missing; a footrest, an armrest or the brake. The ones with faulty wheels don't roll properly or a wheel jams when you go too fast. These chairs are only used for a short time by patients who need them when going from one office to another, or who are waiting for their appointment. The chairs don't need to be well maintained when they are not used much.

There is a little slope on one stretch of the corridor. You can get up quite a speed here. You set off as fast as possible down the slope then see who can roll the furthest in their chair to win.

When the passing uniforms speak to them and, in no uncertain terms, tell them to stop messing about with the wheelchairs, they pretend to stop but, as soon as the uniform disappears around the corner or into the lift, they carry on with their game. The chairs are not being used just now and anyway they are under control. 'Do you think it would be such fun if it was you that had to use it?' they ask. 'We'll put them back when we are finished!' we promise.

A LETTER FROM PAUL

When she gets up to her room she finds a letter on the bed. She can see from the handwriting who it's from. He often writes to her.

Hi Nuts! (ha-ha!)

How's it going?

Things are fine on the whole here.

I've got a game for the Amiga, which is called Platoon.

You've got to lead a troop through the jungles of Vietnam to blow up bridges and things.

We're going to divide the hobby room in the cellar into two with a wall, and I'm getting one of the rooms as a computer room.

I'm now saving up for that Olympic Games game that Atle's got.

So when you come home we can maybe play it.

By the way, Mum's bought you a Barbie magazine, so she'll be sending that soon.

Best wishes from Paul

P.S. I'm not sending you Snap and Crackle sweets this time because you've got to lose weight (according to Mum and Dad). Instead I'm drawing a snap and crackle for you to drool at!

Because she is in hospital for several months she has lessons. The classroom is a table in the corridor outside the children's ward. A screen separates the school from the rest of the corridor. From the world outside.

The screen is a good help in the children's ward. It was white once but there was once a patient with a felt tip pen and nothing to do. That's when these impulsive ideas come. We all know it is easy to carry on something which is already begun and bit by bit the screen has been covered in names and pictures, one on top of another. By the time she has anything to do with the screen it is already over-full. In other words, something to read while you sit in the schoolroom and chew your pencil or use the bedpan in bed.

If you are bed-bound the screen creates the only privacy you get. Privacy in a hospital is when you are using a bedpan, changing bandages, treating a cut, having your temperature measured in your behind, washing or getting dressed and undressed. Every time she is in bed with the screen round because she needs privacy she is nervous in case anyone peeps over it or suddenly come and take it away. 'Can I take this? Oh, sorry. Are you nearly finished?'

The teacher does her best to be understanding but it is not easy to concentrate. She sits behind the screen with the teacher's perfume in her nostrils. The perfume gets stronger when the teacher checks if she has done her maths right. People go by. She listens to their footsteps to see if she recognises them.

Fast or slow?

Short or long strides?

Stomping or light?

Hears two people chatting. She hears them come round the corner. They now are on the other side of the screen. Nurse Reidun is one of them. They have probably been for lunch in the canteen.

'I don't want to be here any longer' she thinks. 'I want to go and play in the play room or listen to a cassette on the Walkman. I want to go down to the ground floor. I want to sit in the nurses' office. I don't want to sit still here!'

'Well done, but you've missed that one and that one is wrong. When you have finished those two we will do some Norwegian.'

Sometimes she tries to escape before the teacher comes and gets her for her lessons. She hides. If the teacher spots her she disappears into the lift or the stairs. Up and down between the floors. The teacher trots after her with her teacher's voice calling 'Little Tweet, Tweety-pie!!'

The teacher calls her Little Tweet or Tweety-pie. It is because of the cage. The teacher thinks it is fun but she thinks it sounds stupid.

The cellar at Aunt and Uncle's in Holmlia has got the Barbie dolls. The exciting Barbies with clothes and furniture that smell and are quite different from those she has at home. She really likes coming here to play, together with Linda. The cellar also has a piano on which she learns to play *Heart and Soul*, that left-hand-and-right-hand song that everyone can play. She learns the simple tune that you use for both hands.

They dress up. She is a wicked witch who has taken a princess prisoner, but the princess is clever and says the opposite of what she really means.

Witch: 'Do you like coffee?'

Princess: 'No!'

Witch: 'Then you have to drink LOTS of coffee! HA, HA!!'

It is Linda who thinks of the princess fooling the witch like this and even though she really ought to be on the witch's side she goes along with the princess's plan. She thinks that everything her cousin thinks up is exciting.

In the ice-cream box is the play-dough. Fingers shape it into princesses, princes and a witch. Heidi and Linda are good at making figures. The princess's hair is long with curls right down her back. The ice-cream box is the castle where the princess stands on the walls and calls out to the prince.

When MTV plays Aunt's favourite song, *If you don't know me by now* with Simply Red, Aunt turns up the volume. When music videos by Guns n Roses and Bon Jovi come on, it is Linda who turns up the volume and the girls stare dreamily at the screen.

She sighs in ecstasy when George Michael, supported by some ropes hanging from the ceiling, looks through the screen and stares into her eyes whilst singing, soft as silk, that he's 'never gonna dance again.'

TV in Oslo is Pat Sharp, Fun Factory, Swedish-language cartoons, Horror Show and music videos. Everything they don't have at home.

Christine comes home from England, bringing a doll each. The doll has long, fair hair and is dressed in a pink and mint-green ballet dress. The doll has make-up which can be removed with cold water and comes back again with warm water.

Uncle gives us prickly goodnight hugs, beard scraping cheeks, and Aunt tells us stories about the terror that lives in the ski slope just across the road and who doesn't like disobedient children. 'But don't tell Linda it's not true' whispers Aunt while Linda is in the bathroom.

One night they are awake until four o'clock, at least. While they others are sleeping, they lie on mattresses in front of the TV in the lounge and watch

Horror Show, with vampires climbing out of their coffins. This is a programme they're not really allowed to watch, but only Heidi sees that they are up so late and she has to promise not to tell tales. Even so, Aunt and Uncle know about it the next day. Perhaps because the two girls are so tired at breakfast time. Aunt has put a milk carton on the breakfast table. The girl reads the words on it and puzzles about them, just as she does every morning at Holmlia.

There are two kinds of Norwegian, two different languages really, and everything is written differently in Oslo from how it is in Sandane. She understands that there are two different languages, but she doesn't see why she can understand everything people say in Oslo, whilst they sometimes ask her to speak Norwegian. Why can't everyone in Oslo understand her? It's just silly, because then she has to speak differently from how she speaks at home, and use different words. Then when she gets home, people at school say that she's begun to talk very posh, but the way they say it makes it sound as though they don't think it's a good thing. So then she has to change the words back again.

Sister Inger Johanne takes her into an empty room with a telephone on a little table. She wonders whether they're going to play a trick on Sister Kari. Sister Kari is in charge, but she's not a strict boss. She messes around and plays jokes just as much as the others, even though sometimes she has to be serious. Inger Johanne wants her to ring the ward and play a joke on Sister Kari. The ward telephone is on Sister Kari's desk and Inger Johanne knows Sister Kari is in there right now. They decide what would be the most believable to say, but when Inger Johanne has finished dialling the number she doesn't dare take the telephone. Inger Hohanne says the trick will work best if it's she who speaks, but she chickens out. Inger Johanne has to speak. 'Some flowers have come to the children's ward,' she says, in a put-on voice, 'can you come down to Reception and collect them now?'

'Inger Johanne?' Sister Kari recognises her voice immediately and Inger Johanne begins to giggle. All three laugh. Luckily Sister Kari isn't cross. She hasn't ever seen Sister Kari cross. Now she regrets that she didn't play the trick. It would have been such fun. She doesn't know what she had been afraid of. She really wanted to be part of the joke. To be the fun, joking little girl who messes about and makes other people laugh out loud.

HANNE'S BIRTHDAY

On Friday she's invited to Hanne's birthday party, which is going to be on the following day. That will mean she can't go to Holmlia that weekend. It is tempting to go to the birthday party. When Aunt Grete comes to collect her, she doesn't dare tell her she's not going with her, that she's chosen to go to a birthday party instead of home with her aunt. One of the nurses has to speak to Aunt Grete. 'Won't you even speak to her?' asks the nurse. But she hides in the staff room. Her aunt is standing in the hallway right outside the office. There are two doors between them. 'No.' 'Your Aunt says it's quite all right for you to go to the birthday, but she'd like to see you before she goes home again.' She shakes her head and stares desperately down at the floor. Her stomach aches with embarrassment and she feels really bad that her aunt has to drive all the way back home without her. She can't see her aunt now.

Just go home and come back next weekend, and it will all be forgotten. Please don't be cross with me. I don't want to be difficult. I just want to go the party.

'Your aunt's gone now. She sends her love and says she'll see you next Friday.' 'Mmm.'

A couple of Hanne's friends come to the party. They have an egg-and-spoon race and they buy buns and cakes with Monopoly money. There's a lot of laughter, and even when her friends wonder about her cage she doesn't think about the children's ward even once. Those thoughts don't pop into her mind again until Inger Johanne is driving her home.

Some years later Inger Johanne tells her that she'd never seen anyone eat so many buns and cakes as she did that day. She'd been across and bought loads more cakes than anyone else.

Since she's such a long way from her own family, a lot of people care about her. Not just the nurses. One of the other girls in her ward has a lot of visits from her family. They start to bring sweets and other treats for her as well. After the girl had gone home from the hospital, they come back one day and visit her after they've been to visit their granddad on the floor above. She is thrilled because it's usually her aunt, uncle and cousins that come to visit her.

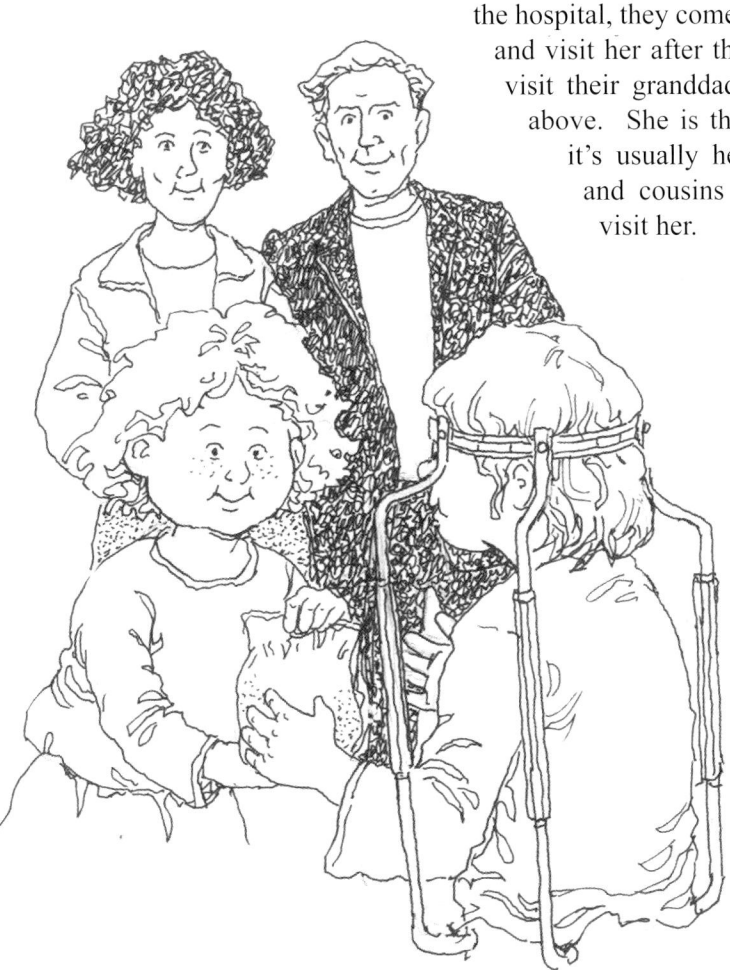

Home sickness is worse at night because that's when her heart is soft and vulnerable. She feels so deserted and alone. She can't keep herself under control like she manages to during the day. And always the same way, and always as bad, whether she's here for six months or one month. She wants her Mum and Dad. She can't pull the duvet up over her head because then she can't breathe. So that none of the others in the room are disturbed and hear her cry she pulls a blanket over and cries silently.

She's been put to bed for the night. The lights in the room are off and the only light comes from the crack under the door. Sometimes the light is broken by the shadows of feet that go to and fro. Her eyes follow the shadows. Will the feet stop outside the room and come in? Are they attached to a body and a smiling face that will come across to her bed and just stay with her until she goes to sleep? But nothing happens.

Do they think of me, the rest of them at home?
Will Mum ring me tomorrow?

The tears start way down in her stomach. She pulls her lips in. A lump works its way up through her chest and up her throat and threatens to burst out. She has to hold it in. The lump sticks in her throat.
You're a brave girl, Anne- Pia.
The pain in her throat, the heavy weight on her chest.
You're really brave.
The pillow's wet but not a sound has come out of her lips through the blanket and into the dark room.

Not a sound… not any other night either.

Sometimes they ask if one or two of the students can help with washing and changing bandages. That's always fine. She can't really be grumpy and say no, because it really doesn't matter, she thinks. And she likes almost all of the student nurses. They spend a bit longer than the qualified nurses. They're enthusiastic to learn, and they ask her why she's here at Sophies Minde hospital. There's one of the students she particularly likes being with, on this her longest visit to the hospital. Torild jokes about everything and laughs a lot. Sometimes she pretends that she's forgotten to have a wash in the ·evening and tries to get away when they come with the bowl. This leads to Torild, with a cheeky smile, starting to call her Grubby-chops. This is a name that she's reminded of long afterwards because Dad gets to know about it.

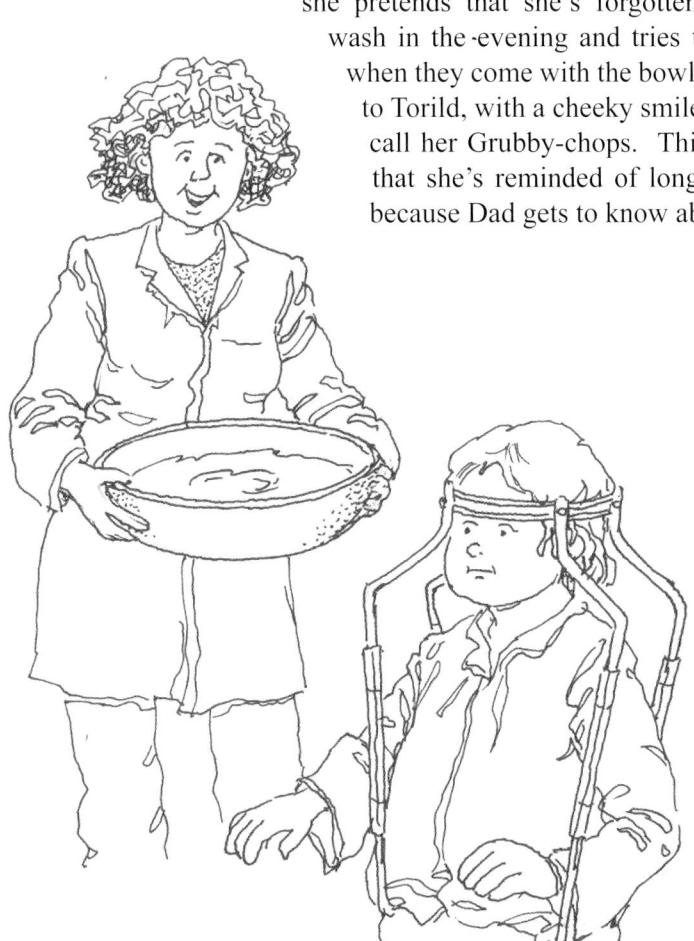

One day she finds out that the hospital management are going to give her 500 kroner to spend on whatever she wants. They sometimes do this for patients who have to spend a very long time in hospital. Torild is going to take her into town shopping, and then they're going to the cinema. She's really looking forward to getting out of the hospital for a while.

Just before they go, she notices the postman has left a massive parcel on her bed. She can see it's come all the way from America and she knows who has sent it; Aunt Eli. In the parcel is a big, soft, pink teddy. She calls it Topsy after Torild's dog. She gives it a big hug, but then it has to wait on her bed until she comes back late in the evening. Because Torild and she are going to town, she explains to Topsy.

Even though it's only a few hours she's thrilled with any time she can be away from the hospital. It's exciting to be allowed out in Oslo. To do things that normal people do. To see things that normal people see every day. All the tall buildings. All the flashing lights as dusk creeps in. The moving pictures on the advertising boards. Buskers singing and making music in the shopping streets. The huge toy shops with row upon row of Barbie dolls and toys – toys that she's only ever seen on TV adverts before. Although Topsy came in the post today she still wants to spend her 500 kroner on a teddy. She chooses a Popples teddy just like the ones on the cartoons on MTV. It's white, with red hair, pink ears, coloured cheeks and can be turned inside out to make a ball.

The cinema shows lots of films at the same time. It's even got its own kiosk and terraced seating, so that you don't have to look at the neck of the person in front of you just because you're smaller than they are.

A man on the train offers her methylated spirit from a bottle from which he's drinking.

DOLL'S PRAM

She spots it on the way out of the playroom. A red doll's pram with a white cover and a pillow with red hearts on. Beside the doll's pram is a man and a lady and Sister Kari. It's not unusual to see people standing in the hallway like this, chatting, so she's a bit surprised when Sister Kari calls her over to where they're standing. At first she thinks they're looking for somebody, but it turns out to be something entirely different. Sister Kari introduces her to the people, tells them her name, her age and how long she's been there. Then she bends down and explains that this man and lady want to give the pram to somebody in the children's ward. They've won it but have decided to give it to somebody who will have more pleasure from it. Sister Kari has said she thinks she ought to get it.

She doesn't realise at first what Sister Kari has just said. It's great that the children's ward are going to get it, she thinks. And then she realises it's her. She's thrilled. She goes over and touches it, rocks it. It stands beside her bed at night. She can see the pale material in the dark. She stretches out a hand to touch it. Gives it a little poke so that it rocks. She thinks of the dolls at home. Which one will be allowed to sleep in it?

Inger Johanne has been on holiday to Copenhagen. Copenhagen is far, far away. The name sounds exotic. Somewhere out there in the world. Somewhere people go on holiday and come back with lots to tell about fairgrounds, shops and red sausages.

She can't point Copenhagen out on a map. She only knows where Sandane is and where Oslo is. She draws a line with her finger from the top and diagonally to the bottom. *This is how far we fly when I have to come to Oslo.*

But Copenhagen is off the map. Beyond anything she knows. Beyond anything she can recognise. Perhaps one day she'll be able to go somewhere like that.

Inger Johanne brings her a present back from her holiday in Copenhagen. A little pink box with a sleeping cat's head on the top. She explains that they speak Danish in Copenhagen.

Imagine, Inger Johanne has thought of her when she was in Copenhagen!

Amongst all the people, all the fun things to see and do over there, she stopped, went across, bent down at a shelf and said 'I'm going to buy that for little Anne-Pia.' A box from Copenhagen.

There's just enough room in it for a penny.

BANDAGES AND STITCHES

Wednesday 13 March 1985

Had an operation at Ullevoll hospital. They put two iron rods in my back.

They've opened my back to put in two iron rods. The bandages which cover the cuts where they operated have to be changed often and it hurts so much. She knows exactly when the nurses are going to change the bandages and she hides. The glue sticks tight to the skin. 'Can't it just stay on?' she begs.

But the nurses work out how to do it. In the morning or evening they loosen the ties on her gown. The gowns are specially made. They have splits up the sides and the back, just in the right place for the rods of the cage to come through. The gown is fastened with laces for every split and you put it on from the back. Every morning and evening she turns her back towards the nurses so they can fasten the gown. They suddenly get hold of one of the corners of the dressing and pull it off before she has time to react. She screams, but actually the worst is over and there's no more pain for the time being.

When they're going to take the stitches out this hurts too, but that's only after each operation and not every day, as it is with the dressings. The nurses say they can count the stitches together, and keep them safe so that she can show them to her friends when she gets back home. They are removed one by one from her back with tweezers and put carefully onto a piece of paper. When they've all been removed there are two rows on the piece of paper and they cover them with a piece of tape. Thirty-one stitches in all.

The post room has cassettes that you can record onto, and send like letters. When she gets audio letters from home, she sits on her bed with the cassette and plays it through a Walkman. It's the red Walkman, the one that falls on the floor every time a nurse tidies up or moves anything on her

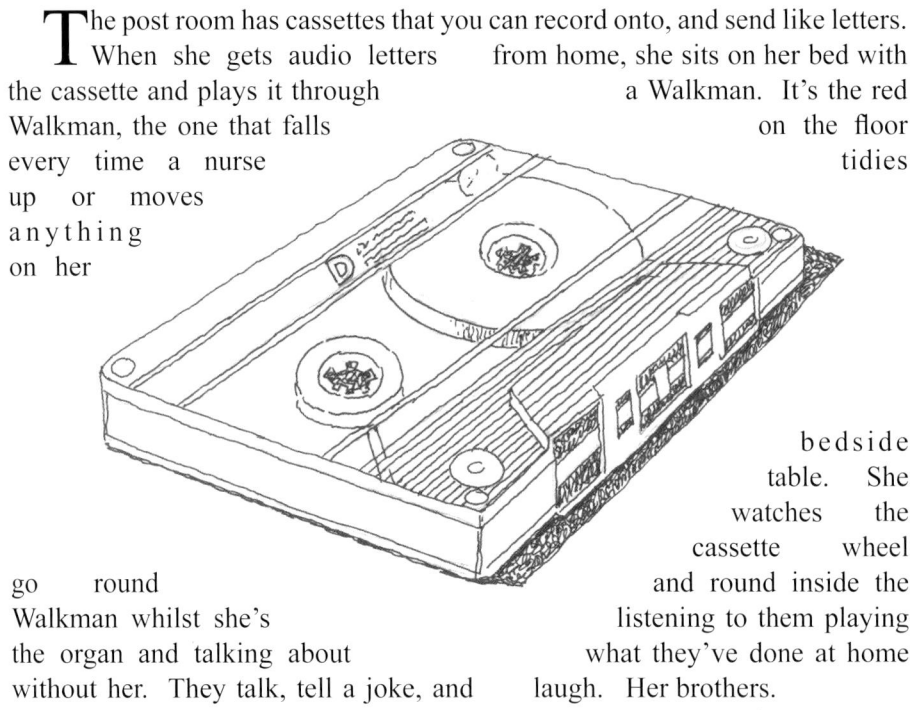

bedside table. She watches the cassette wheel go round and round inside the Walkman whilst she's listening to them playing the organ and talking about what they've done at home without her. They talk, tell a joke, and laugh. Her brothers.

Guro's too little to say anything. *Do you want to say something to Anne-Pia?* She closes her eyes and sees the owners of the voices she can hear. Suddenly she's there, she's with them. They're there, going round and round in the cassette.

FOOD TROLLEY

Her tummy tells her when it's getting near. Not always because she's hungry, but if she is, then the hunger mixes with the other. The expectation. The day's high point. The grey, metallic, food trolley arrives. It's parked beside the nurses' station. It feels like it's there for ever, until eventually the nurses start going round. It's already time – get on with it! Into a room, sitting down, wait. Wait until they come. They always start furthest in, at the other end. When she moves her bed to room 208 because she was friends with someone in that room, she gets her food before room 210. But the disadvantage is that she's also finished earlier. There isn't enough for more than one helping each.

At last the nurses are serving her.

'How much do you want?' 'Is that enough?'

'Yes, that's fine, or ... maybe a bit more?'

A lot of people might say that fish, especially hospital fish, is enough to make you lose your appetite. But not her. The only place she draws the line at is liver. Otherwise she'll eat anything. And if she doesn't she can always sneak down to the chocolate machine afterwards.

She doesn't always have to go far to find chocolate, either. It's only a matter of putting her hand in the drawer of a bedside table. Sometimes she gets sweets in the post from people who know her family and think it's a shame for her, and hope that she'll soon be fully well and can come home again.

Room 210 is decorated for the Eurovision feast. Both the nurses and the patients are in a good mood all day and are looking forward to the high point of the year. The father of one of the other girls has brought enough pizza for everyone. Some people have got a flag in their hand. And the atmosphere is great. 'This time it's our turn to win, or at least we have to beat the Swedish as they're at home.' 'Listen to what the Turkish song is called – *didai didai dai*.'

'Or Portugal – *Penso em ti, eu sei.*'

'What about Cyprus, then? – *To katalava aga.*'

'Can't pronounce the title of the Greek song – *Moiazoume.*'

The Norwegian contestants come confidently onto the stage dressed in black, with glittering lilac jackets. The song is catchy and easy to sing along to.

Let it swing and let it rock and roll
Let it swing and let the feeling take control.

Before the competition has got as far as the scoring, her eyes are so heavy and her back is so weary that she just wants to go to bed. It doesn't feel like long from when she drops off to sleep with music in the background and chatting in the room, until she wakes to happy faces and voices. 'Good morning. Wake up! Guess what? Norway won! At last we've won the Eurovision Song Contest!'

Marianne is blind and uses a wheelchair to help her. She's always happy and playing tricks. And others play along with her when really they don't dare. Marianne allies herself with her and, because she doesn't want to be a wimp, she ends up filling a bucket with water while Marianne gets somebody tall to put it on top of the door to the nurses' office. Another time they get hold of some sheets and play ghosts in borrowed wheelchairs.

Once, when there's only the two of them in the room, Marianne has a fit. She's thrown back in the wheelchair. Her eyes roll into her head and she foams at the mouth. She's petrified when she sees this happen to Marianne. She's never seen anything like that happen before and she doesn't know what to do. Fortunately the nurses are quickly on the scene. Marianne's had a serious epileptic fit. She slowly comes round. And is soon happy again, as though nothing has happened.

A year later, at an outpatient appointment, the nurse asks if she knows about Marianne. She is confused. 'What do you mean?' Of course she knows who Marianne is. They used to play together. She answers carefully because she doesn't quite know where the conversation is going. She goes into the playroom and waits for the doctor, while her Dad sits in the hallway and waits. Some people are sitting, drawing at a table. Eli, who is in charge of the playroom and used to take me outside to the play area, is talking to some adults.

'Oh, it was dreadful, what happened to Marianne'. She pricks her ears up.

'What?' Eli tells her that Marianne died of a heart attack not long ago.

'Didn't you know?'

It's unbelievable. Marianne was so alive, so mischievous. She can't imagine her dead.

24 April 1985

They took the cage off

After four months the cage was surgically removed. She's been screwed 8cm taller and the curvature in her spine has been straightened out. Now she needs a Boston corset again. The corset has to stay on all day so that her spine is supported. They take a plaster cast of her body and from that make a corset with ventilation in the stomach and an opening at the back that can be tightened with straps. It runs from under her arms to beyond her hips. Between the corset and her skin is a big piece of cloth to make it more comfortable.

Departure day has arrived. Her bags are packed by her bed and she's waiting impatiently for Dad who's coming by plane to collect her. She thinks that when he goes home she'll be going with him. She won't be left behind with a lump in her throat and a feeling of being forgotten. This time, it's going to be her that turns and waves goodbye to all those people she's got to know between the white walls in the big room. The nurses tease her that now it's almost 17 May. *Doesn't she want to stay a little bit longer so that she can go in the national day procession and wave at the King?* But she just wants to go home. Nothing would convince her to stay any longer.

She's waiting in the playroom when a smiling nurse comes in and says, 'Dad's arrived now.' Behind the nurse is a familiar face and she feels like the whole world must see that it's her Dad come to take her home. She almost can't believe that he really is standing there and he's not just in her imagination like so many times before. The whole situation seems odd and unlikely, but she's happy and everything is magical.

At the same time, in Sandane, a ten-year-old lad is standing in front of a long table made up of several tables next to each other. It's a jumble sale. Lots of jumble in rows and piles are being picked up and put down again. The ten-year-old stands there and carefully studies the things on the table. He doesn't really know what he wants, but he'll know it when he sees it. Esther, who's behind one of the tables, notices him and recognises him.

'Are you going to buy something nice today, Paul?', she asks.

'It's not for me', replies the boy, 'it's for Anne-Pia. She's coming home from the hospital'.

Esther notices the pride in his voice. He's the big brother who's going to buy something nice for his little sister. He's a very happy young man with money in his hand. Esther notices the excitement in his eyes. It's obvious there's something he's looking forward to.

'Really? That's good news. And how lovely that you're buying her a present.'

The young man has found something that he's now considering. It's an old-fashioned brown bag with press-studs and a lot of pockets.

'How much is this?' he asks.

'Oh, I don't want more than two kroner for that,' says Esther, and smiles.

Paul gives the money to the nice lady behind the table, takes the bag and goes home.

When Guro was born she'd been looking forward to it for a long time. 'It might be a girl.' And it was. No-one was more proud than herself. She got up early to watch when Mum was washing and caring for Guro and she loved cuddling and playing with. Yes, having a little sister was great. But… now Guro was a bit bigger, her thoughts did wander towards the idea that being an only girl had meant that she could have her dolls in peace. Neither Paul nor Peter had really invaded her territory or disturbed her things.

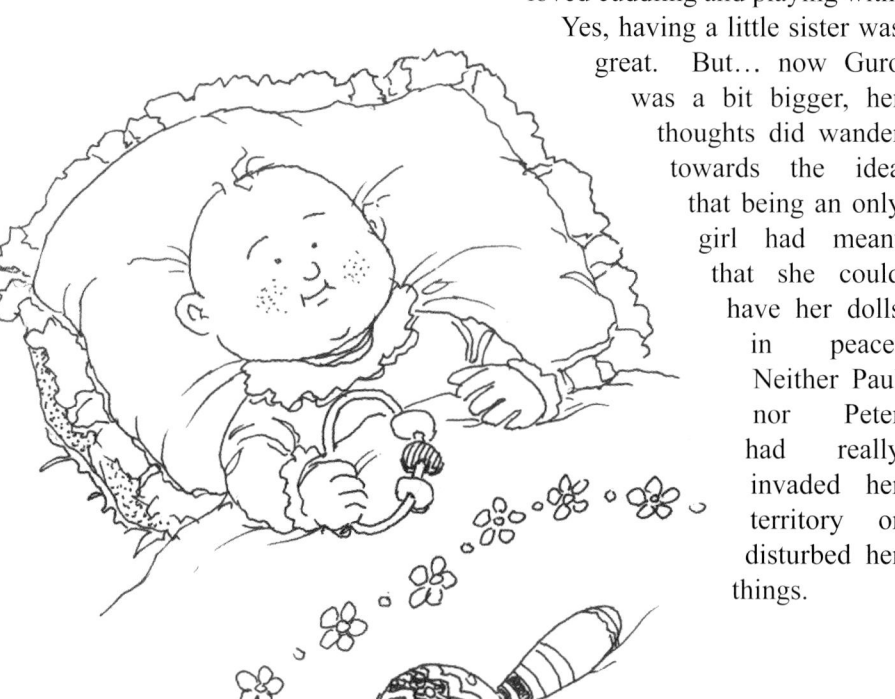

Her back is still quite weak and she's not allowed to run or lift anything heavy. This is immediately after six months in the hospital. The saddest part about it is that she can't carry Guro. Disobeying the doctors never enters her head. She doesn't want anything to go wrong.

But something happens that she keeps to herself. In the kitchen, Guro has clambered up onto a chair and is crying because she can't get down again. There's only the two of them there and, without thinking about it, she puts her arms around the baby and lifts her safely down onto the floor again. It happens so fast. The crying stopped and she realises she shouldn't have done that. But something that was so quick surely couldn't have done any damage?

She receives home education for the first month because of her weak back, and she has to lie down for the lessons. A special writing board is made to go over her, so that she can do her work. Her bed in her bedroom can be turned into a sofa, and this is where her classroom is. She does her maths lying down while her teacher sits beside her, reading Donald Duck comic books.

Taxi

Once the home education ended, she had to go and come back from school in a taxi. In the beginning, she lay across the back seat as they drove, but after a while she was allowed to sit normally.

Every day had been difficult for the first three years of school. By the time she got home she was exhausted and threw herself on the sofa. She'd had trouble keeping up with Ragnhild, whom she walked with, and sometimes she suddenly had to go to the toilet when they were only half way. It never occurred to anybody that she might have a claim for transport to and from school. But after that last operation nobody mentioned her walking to school any more.

The following summer, Mum goes along with her back to the hospital for more investigations and measurements for a new corset. Mum's going to stay with her whilst she's an inpatient.

Crown Princess Martha's Institute, where her mother is going to stay, is next door to Sophies Minde hospital. Here they are self-catering, which means that one doesn't feel as closed in and restrained as in a hospital. During the day it's almost possible to forget the reason they're in Oslo. It's summer, the sky is blue, and the sun shines all the time. It's like being on holiday.

They get to know another mother and daughter. The mother is also staying at the Institute, while the daughter is with Anne-Pia in room 210. The girl is a couple of years older and also uses a corset. They become good friends and find things to fill their days. Mum has got someone to talk and knit with, and the girls chat and go across to the fruit and tobacco kiosk on the corner, which also sells sweets and comics. Mum buys her a white summer dress with a picture of an Indian on the front and long fringes. For Guro, who has just had her second birthday, they buy a nightdress with an elephant on. When they have to be in the hospital waiting for the doctor, it doesn't matter because she knows that, even if she wanders round in the hallways or the playroom, Mum's in her room, knitting. She only has to go back to her room and there's Mum.

Every morning she wakes with a big smile because Mum's not far away. She'll soon be with her, right until bed time.

And so the week passes.

DIARY NOTES 1

Wednesday 27 August 1986

Dear Diary,

Today we've got swimming at school. I'm allowed to swim as well. Ragnhild helps me take my corset off and a teacher helps me put it back on.

4 November 1986

Dear Diary,

Today I'm an inpatient at Sophies Minde hospital again. Dad and I flew here. We were in the air for two hours twenty minutes.

Sunday 14 December 1986

Dear Diary,

I've been operated on, again. This is my fifth operation. I went to the hospital on 4 November and was there for one month and one week. Bjerkreim (the doctor) said that one of the rods in my back has loosened so I have to take it easy. He said it might fix itself, but if it if it doesn't fix itself I'm going to have to have another operation and I don't want to. They're going to cut in at the side if I need another operation. I dread another operation. I hope I don't need one.

Yours,
A-P N.

3 January 1987

Psst! it's corrected itself!

Saturday 21 February 1987

Dear Diary,

I am fed up with Guro going in my room.
Today I said I was going to go and make a mess in her room. But I didn't.
Guro thought I did and told Peter. And Peter thought I had. Really it was Guro who'd made a mess in her room the day before. Peter went into her room and saw the mess.
I got the blame. I was really unlucky and they told me off and I was innocent.
They're standing by my door, still telling me off and I'm writing my diary in my room. What a day, eh?

Best wishes

Psst they're going to ring the police.

Thursday 12 march 1987

Dear Diary,

Dad and I are going to an outpatient appointment at the hospital in Oslo today. Wish me luck.
Mum's bought me a Donald Duck comic book and a packet of biscuits.

Friday 13 March 1987

Dear Diary,

Everything was fine. The doctors were satisfied with my back. I'm now allowed to sit in a car and I can start school on Monday.

Yours truly, Anne-Pia

Half past eleven in the morning.

Tuesday 17 March 1987

Dear Diary,

Yesterday I went to school. It went fine, except that …
I FELL.
The doctors said that I mustn't run, mustn't cycle and mustn't… fall.
But I did.
I've got an outpatients appointment in six months, so don't tell mum that I fell. I've not told her. If everything is fine I will tell her.

Yours, Anne-Pia.

Sunday 9 August 1987

Dear Diary,

It's my birthday tomorrow and I hope it's nice weather.
Dad offended me today by saying I'd put on weight. I'm trying as hard as I can. I just can't do it. It's like being a failure of a child.
Oh well. I'll just have to live with it.

Goodbye, best wishes,
Yours, Anne-Pia.

Friday 4 September 1987

Dear Diary,

Yesterday, Mum and I went to see a road they're making. When we'd gone along it a bit we came to a place where they were going to use explosives. I panicked and dragged Mum with me up a side road and covered our ears. As we walked along we came to a forest and we picked and ate blueberries.

Luckily we got home, but we thought we'd got lost.

Sunday 6 September 1987

Dear Diary,

On Friday I was at school as usual with Janne and after school I asked the taxi to drive up to Janne because we'd arranged it. I stayed over and when I came home on Saturday I was going to a birthday party. The night I slept at Janne's and we told
ghost stories.

Yours truly, Anne-Pia

Monday 5 October 1987

Dear Diary,

Quite a few days ago I had the flu. Now I've got an infection in a cut on my foot. I've had flu twice. My foot hurts so much I have to lie down almost all day. But today, Peter, Gran and I went to the doctor. Peter's got... uhh, I can't remember what it's called. It's a type of rash or something. I've got to take Pastlin tablets (or something like that).

Gran bought some new shoes for me today. They wanted to throw the old ones away but I saved them. I 'smuggled' them into my room without anybody noticing. That's what I call smart.

Yours Anne-Pia

To Utvik mountain on a dog-sleigh

We've got a happy mother on the line.

'We have a daughter who, due to her illness, can't take part in playground games and sports activities in her free time,' says Turid Nygård, 'This also means that she's not been able to go on skis this winter.

'But last weekend, Anne-Pia had an unforgettable experience on Utvik mountain. Anders Hole took the initiative which enabled her to go with Magne Solheim from Gloppen Dog club and Nordleif Jordanger from Breim on a sleigh trip. This was a new and exciting treat for Anne-Pia and her siblings and I'm very grateful to those who made it possible', says Turid Nygård.

'They absolutely deserve a thanks in this paper'.

Some time after the last operation she's allowed to be more active. Back at school after her most recent trip to Oslo she's really pleased because the doctors have said that she's allowed to run again! At last she can join in properly with the games at playtime. Ragnhild joins her in running round and round and round the playground in celebration. Now she can play hopscotch and skipping and rounders and dodgeball. She can start to be normal, just like all the others.

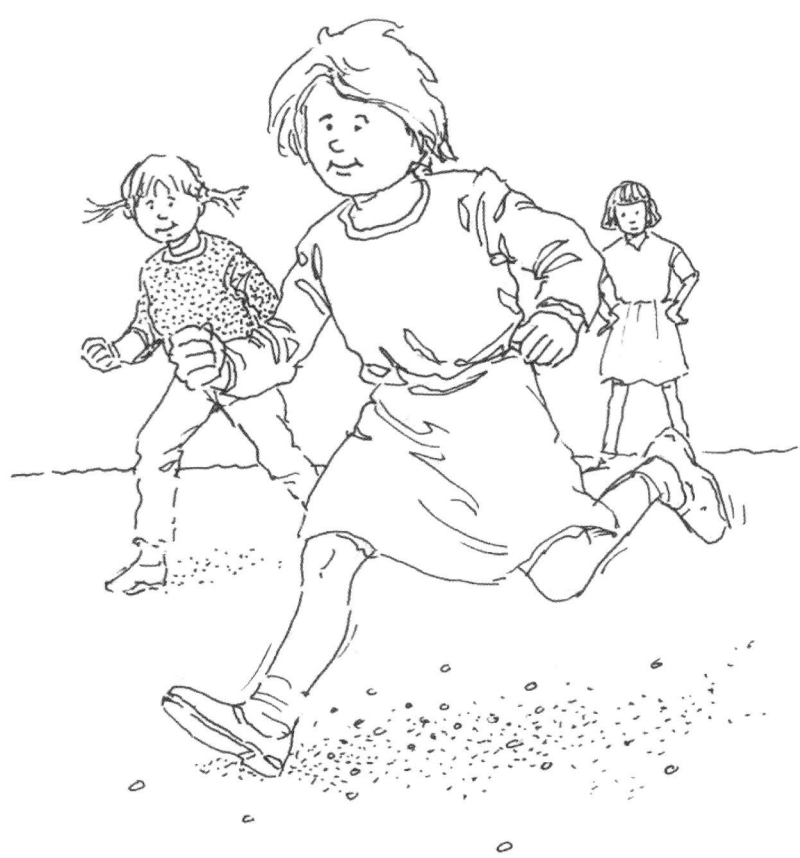

DIARY NOTES 2

Saturday 7 November 1987

Dear Diary,

Today is sad and I'm cross. Mum was at work and Dad was at home and he didn't go into Sandane so we didn't get any crisps for with children's TV this evening. I'm sad and fed up and cross and angry, as Mum calls it.
Yesterday was fun. I went to an Indian party and afterwards to a bazaar.

Sunday 13 December 1987

Dear Diary,

It's nearly Christmas!
Yesterday we made ginger biscuits. Yesterday I joined the 4H youth club. I chose the 'mini-carpenter' group. Ragnhild is starting her second year in the 4H club. Ragnhild, Lillian, Hildegunn and I chose 'mini-carpenter'. Ragnhild and I are in the same group.
It is fun.

Yours,
Anne-Pia

You can't fail to notice that her legs are letting her down. But she's just been allowed to stop using the corset, so it's not surprising that the muscles in her body, especially in her back, are weak after years of using a corset, and that affects the legs. But the fact is that, more and more often, her legs aren't always with her. Mum and Dad tell her off because she trips and doesn't manage to walk properly. She's already had to be re-operated on twice. The rods had to be changed for new ones because they were broken.

In autumn 1987, Doctor Haga sends a letter to Sophies Minde Hospital explaining the deterioration and asking for an outpatients appointment:

'An increased tendency to trip over her toes and fall... She has evident weakness in her lower extremities and it is possible that she could gain better control of her body and lessen her tendency to fall by physiotherapy on her lower extremities. I do not wish to begin this as I don't know what consequences it might have for her back. I ask that you review it with a view to active physiotherapy to strengthen and train her leg muscles. As you know, there are significant other problems in addition to those in her back, and perhaps it would be best if she was taken into hospital in September instead of just having an outpatients appointment. I presume you will consider this.'

Two months after that letter was sent she is called to an outpatients appointment at Sophies Minde Hospital but the doctors cannot find anything of concern. In her hospital records the doctor writes that there are no complications after the operation. Everything appears to be stable and he can find no neurological reason for her tripping. He advises physiotherapy to increase strength and coordination and a follow-up appointment in six months.

THE LAST CHRISTMAS THAT SHE CAN WALK

It's Christmas. As usual the day started with Disney cartoons, then a visit to her grandparents where they had burgers and hot chocolate and exchanged gifts. They're allowed to open one small present each when they come home, then they change into their best clothes.

After Christmas dinner and a rest on the sofa for the adults, it's present time. Again Dad tells the story of when Peter was small and sneaked in to see which presents were his so that he 'by accident' found all of his first, but then screamed his head off whilst all the others were getting theirs and there were no more left for him. That Christmas she can't face getting up off the settee so often so the others get her presents for her.

When Father Christmas turns up, later that evening, she manages to go across the floor for the obligatory Father Christmas picture. She's always been afraid of him, never felt quite safe with this stranger who comes into their sitting room at Christmas, the finest time of the year. But her suspicion vanishes and is replaced with a little less suspicion when she realised that it was Dad's skin and Dad's throat that was sticking out from under the mask and beard. *It's only Dad!*, she thought in surprise, and tried to point this out to Paul. Whether he'd already discovered this for himself or whether he just didn't care because he was busy with his new building set is difficult to know. Even though Dad's secret is now out she still doesn't feel relaxed and natural around him, but Father Christmas belongs to Christmas and out onto the floor she has to go, despite fear and her legs making her reluctant.

Her legs have deteriorated over the winter and in the end she has had enough; she lies on the sofa all day. When she needs to go to the toilet she stands on her Dad's feet and he walks for her.

On New Year's Eve Dad rings Dr Haga. Mum and Dad are worried. Haga gets in touch with the hospital again, this time by telephone. She is told she can come the following week.

That evening she goes out around the village with the other children, dressed up and collecting sweets from the neighbours, a Norwegian tradition repeated all over the country at this time of year. They visit a couple of houses before she decides to wait at the top of a steep hill whilst the others go down to the terraced houses. Eventually she sees them heading back up the hill but, instead of coming all the way up to her, they go into Ragnhild and Eystein's house, where they've already been She can't face following them and goes home crying. It's a disappointment not to be able to join in. A feeling of being alone hits her.

Before most people are properly awake, have wiped the sleep out of their eyes and got themselves to work or to school, father and daughter are climbing out of the plane in Oslo. But this time there's no time for them to wait for her to walk slowly. Dad picks her up and carries her on his back. This time she can't make her legs move fast enough. At the hospital they borrow a wheelchair for her to sit in while they're waiting for the X-ray department.

Sister Kari walks past the doorway to the waiting room. Sister Kari is one of her favourite nurses. She's always pleased to see her and smiles with pleasure. Sister Kari looks very surprised and wonders what they are doing here. Then Sister Kari spots the wheelchair. Used as she is to patients using wheelchairs unnecessarily, she's still surprised. The girl explains that something is wrong with her legs and she can barely stand up without holding onto something. She can't even manage to walk across the hall, and that's why they're here. Nurse Kari's hand moves automatically to her heart. 'I had no idea,' she says sadly.

Suddenly everything is more serious now that Sister Kari, who always smiles and laughs, has a serious look on her face. Her sorrow makes an impression on me. It's not that I don't realise that something is wrong, but thought that everything would be fine. I don't want to be like this any longer. I don't want the pain. I don't want to have suddenly to run to the toilet. I don't want to be embarrassed about myself, feel guilty because I can't even walk properly. And of course Dr Long can help. He'll make everything better. I also hope Dad thinks we've got time to visit the children's ward before it's time to go again.

In the doctor's office, she has to see a different doctor since Dr Lange is in the middle of an operation. A new, unknown doctor. The new doctor hangs up the X-ray pictures and says he can't see anything wrong.

'But there must be something that isn't as it should be, when I have to carry her in!' says a worried Dad.

'The only problem I can see is that her muscles are weak and they need to be trained. I can see no reason to do anything before her next outpatient's appointment in six months' time.'

In the doctor's notes he writes:

'Patient attends outpatient's appointment. Since she was here last she has become noticeably less steady. She cannot walk without supporting herself. It appears that she has developed weak legs… X-rays taken today do not appear to show any change in her back or with the Harrington Staves. An application should be made to the children's ward in the National Hospital for further investigations by neurological specialists.'

W̲hen she gets back from Oslo on 9 January 1988 with her Dad, she goes straight to her pink bean bag. Her legs are extremely tired and she wants to rest.

That transpires to be her very last step.

She has to be lifted up from the bean bag. Her legs will no longer carry her, nor has she any feeling in them.

Note from the little blue diary:

I am lame. Me, Mum and Dad are going to Oslo. Sophies Minde Hospital.

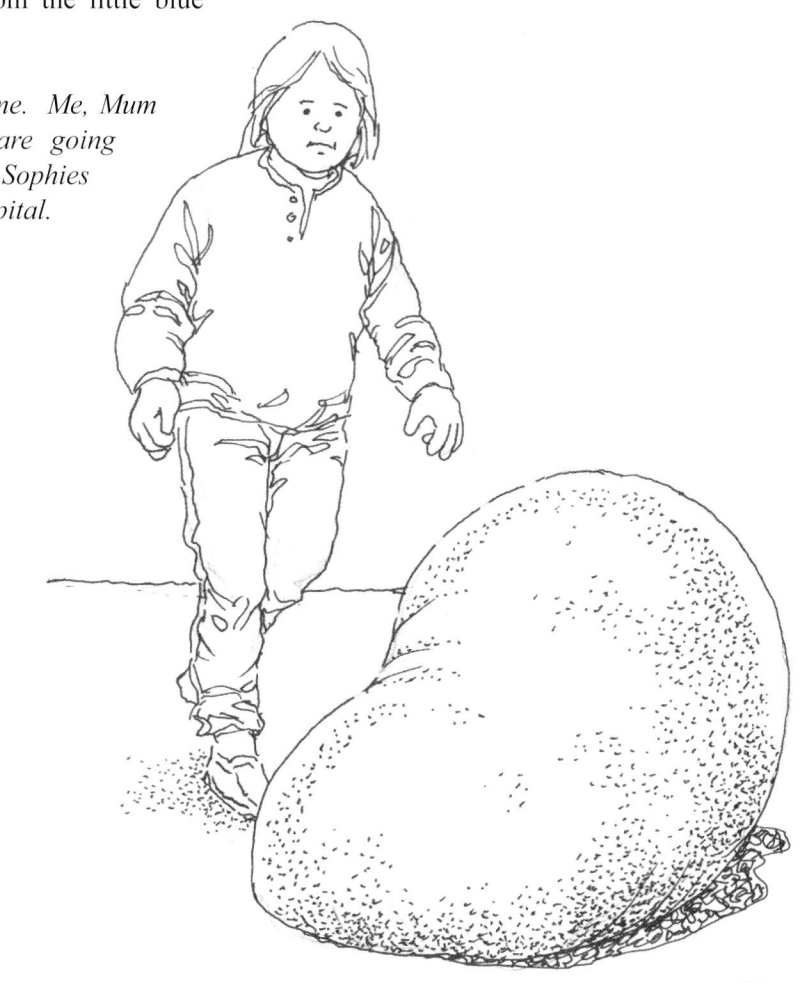

Doctor Haga immediately contacts Sophies Minde who for once act quickly. A sample of spinal fluid is taken and then she is immediately moved across to the National Hospital. The National Hospital take X-rays and when they read them they can immediately see that something is wrong.

When Mum and Dad come with her to the National Hospital, all the staff know that this is the girl that has been wrongly diagnosed. Everybody is affected by the story and one of the doctors says in a worried voice to Dad, 'If only you'd come straight here!'

'Well, we would have if we'd been allowed to,' said Dad.

The doctor continues: 'A couple of days sooner and we could have fixed this without any problem but now the chances are minimal.'

After she's been given medication to help her relax, one of the staff reads her a story before she falls asleep. The operation the following day reveals that her spinal cord is completely squashed by one of the Harrington Staves, both of which are broken. This time they put in a new stave and an iron plate.

Sophies Minde is ready to receive her when she's moved across. Dad has to go home early and, not many days later, Mum has to go too. Mum sits and cries during the flight and when eventually the plane lands at Sandane airport Mum rushes out to the waiting car. She doesn't glance up at all so that she doesn't have to meet the curious eyes of those around her. 'Mum, why are you crying?' ask the three children who've come to collect her from the airport.

Thursday 28 January 1988

Dear Diary,

It started last summer: my legs failed me. I can't walk any more.
Now I'm lying in bed in room 210, reading. I've had another operation on my back. The stitches are out, I've got a corset. I sit in a wheelchair now and then.
Nurse Kari and I bet 10 kroner on when I'd get my corset. I won (of course).

Yours,
Anne-Pia

Sunday 31 January 1988

Dear Diary,

Today I have been in my wheelchair almost all day.
Nurse Aase broke a glass into at least a thousand pieces.
Cathrine came to visit today. On Tuesday Dad's coming down.
A couple of days ago I/we hoisted a nurse (Inger Johanne) up in a bed.
Otherwise everything as usual.

Yours Anne-Pia

There is a hope that the paralysis will improve, but the prognosis is not good.

In the blue diary from the local savings bank she writes:

2 February, Tuesday

Dad came.

5 February

Dad went.

We ate porridge in room 210. Inger Johanne thought that was good.

Saturday

Was in the standing frame. The string broke.

Sunday

Aunt was here.

Monday

Mum rang. Have been given a challenge to draw 210 and what happens there. Wash my hair.

Because of the paralysis she has no control over her bladder. To strengthen that muscle, so that she avoids having to empty her bladder with a catheter, they try a method whereby every couple of hours, when her bladder has filled itself, it is gently banged until it automatically empties. She is laid on the bed with the bedpan underneath and eventually learns how to knock and press her bladder gently. She has to lie like this until she is sure that her bladder is properly empty.

One morning she is lying tapping her bladder with the bedpan underneath and meanwhile the nurse goes to do something else. The sister has put the curtains around the bed but forgotten to cover her lower body with a blanket or cover. She ought to have said something to the nurse but she didn't like to, even though she felt uncomfortable lying there half naked. She is convinced that she whinges too much. It's the same feeling that she has when she rings the bell and asks for help. She's always afraid of asking for too much or disturbing them. *It doesn't matter if I have to lie like this for a little bit until she comes back and realises what she's forgotten.*

New sounds in the room. A group of doctors has come in. Fortunately they head over to one of the other patients, but then suddenly one of the doctors peeps over the curtains to where she's lying. He can see how she's lying there, but even so he doesn't avert his eyes. She feels very uncomfortable and doesn't know what to do or whether she should say something to him. It feels like he stands there for a long time but never meets her eyes. She's frozen in that position. She doesn't know whether her hand is still pressing or has stopped. Eventually he disappears behind the curtain.

Nobody gets to know about this episode, because what is there to tell? That doctor often comes into the room because he is the allocated doctor for Elin in the next bed. Elin often talks about him and laughs with him when he's there. But even though she's often with them it's as though he doesn't see her. She's stupid to expect he'll say anything, an apology or anything. He doesn't say anything, neither one thing nor another. It's as though it never happened, and she keeps quiet. She certainly can't say anything to Elin because Elin really likes him.

Some of the nurses take a group of them from the ward to the circus. Hanne comes too. Also Frode, who's had surgery on his back. He's a two-metre-high, sixteen-year-old with a corset. Hanne and she sit right at the front, near where the animals are kept, since that's the only place she can sit with a wheelchair. The others have tickets right at the back.

During the show the public are encouraged to come forward to try to ride a horse at the gallop without falling off. Immediately, a long thin shape comes down towards the stables. Frode's going to try. She and Hanne talk excitedly and almost can't believe their eyes. But when they begin to fasten Frode into the safety harness the excitement jumps to another level as Hanne shouts 'Mum's coming!' And, quite right, Inger Johanne is heading into the area at full speed to stop Frode.

But the ringmaster misunderstands and thinks she also wants to try riding. Before Inger Johanne can explain the misunderstanding she too is fastened into a safety harness. Round and round the ring gallop Frode and Inger Johanne on their horses. The look on their faces! The one enthusiastic and happy; Inger Johanne just petrified. And it doesn't take many minutes, or perhaps it's only seconds, before Inger Johanne and Frode are thrown off, to the wild excitement of the public.

He came with something for you. It's on your bedside table.'
She looks curiously at the nurse. *What's all this about? Has he got something for me? Does he like me?* She can feel herself start to blush and hurries into her room. *How on earth can I face him after that? It's so embarrassing if he's fallen in love with me. What if the others tease me?*

At first she can't see anything. *Is it a letter, or a note? Oh, I wonder what he's written...* Then she notices something that wasn't there before – a piece of cloth. That's what's popular in the playroom at the moment – painting on cloth. *Has he made something for me? How exciting!*

She picks it up and unfolds it. It looks familiar. She's made something very similar. She looks at it more closely. It is hers. She forgot it in the playroom. She realises now. Her heart falls heavily back into position and she realises he's just been asked to give it to her.

I suppose that's fine, she thinks and looks around her slightly embarrassed. *What was I thinking of?*

She goes down to the activity room quite often, to make things, or into the ward playroom where Ingunn the play therapist is. It's difficult to understand Ingunn sometimes, because she's from Sogndal. Sogndal isn't far away but the dialect is very different. As they get to know each other, and she's allowed to go home with Ingunn to have barbeques, it becomes easier to understand her. She likes white cheese so much she even teaches Ingunn to put it in her salad, like her Mum had always done.

The hospital caretaker helps her build a house for her Barbie dolls. It has four rooms and a stable. She's even allowed wallpaper paste in her room so that she can decorate it herself. She paints the outside in Barbie pink.

Physiotherapy means stretching her legs so that the paralysed joints don't stiffen. It's very important that her joints remain supple so that it's not difficult to get dressed. Training her upper body and arms is of course a very important part of her routine, so that she will become as strong and independent as possible.

A good routine for toileting is another important task. When they realised that the paralysis would not improve, they didn't continue the tapping of her bladder. To be sure that her bladder was emptied she now has to catheterise herself every five hours. That means weeing through a tube. The catheter is threaded in through her urinary tract and, even though it's neither painful nor unpleasant, it is probably one of the most difficult things to get used to doing. She has no desire whatsoever to learn to do it, so the tuition is postponed until the Autumn when she's going to Sunnaas Rehabilitation Hospital for more training.

A SHORT VISIT HOME

It's March. Mum and Dad come to bring her home. She's allowed on a home visit for a couple of weeks before going back to Oslo. Home education has been arranged this time at the kitchen table.

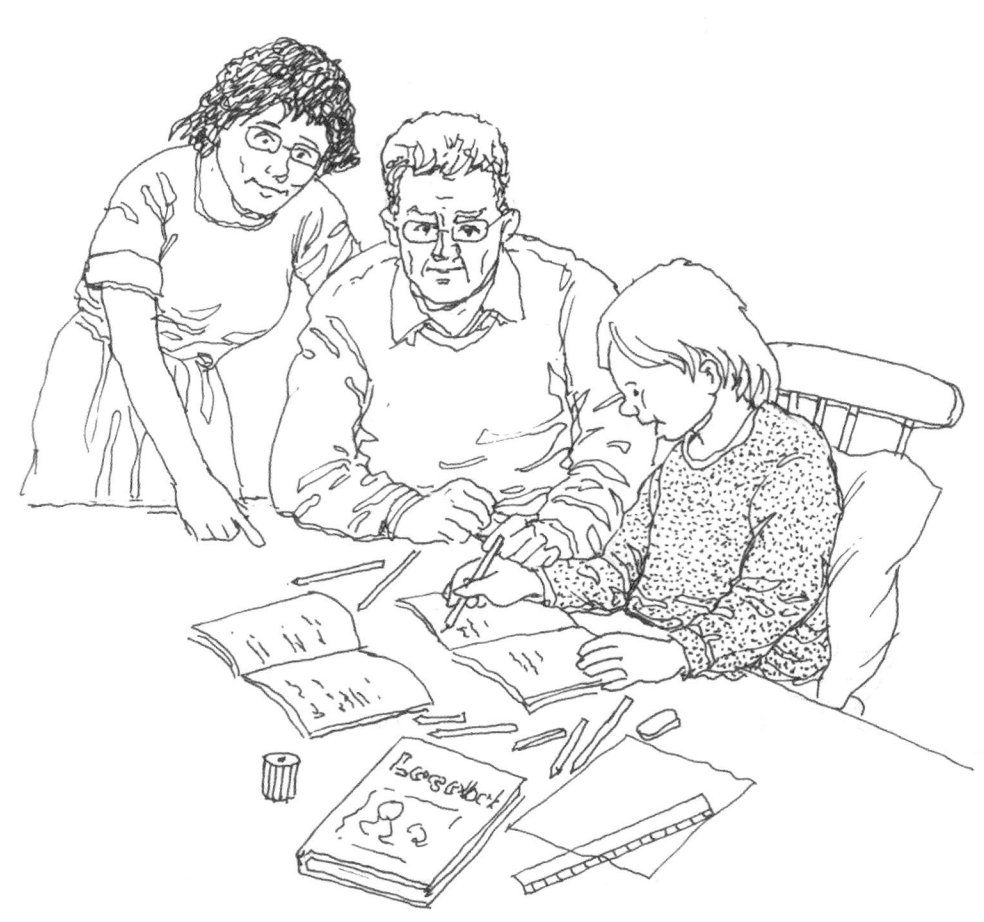

Sophies Minde – 88

Dear Anne Pia

I will never
Forget you,
Even though you won't remember me.
First you had a cage on,
But you never got a rage on.
Now you use a wheelchair,
Yet you smile as if you haven't a care.
There is only one Anne- Pia
In the world.

Best wishes, Kari.

Greetings to Anne Pia

Hip hip hurra
Anne- Pia's heading home.
And we won't get told off
any more
– or called names!

But the sun is shining and
Pia is glowing
Because away from
'Minde' she now is going.

Hugs from Reidun

Dear Anne-Pia,

'Allo, 'allo, Anne!
I'm trying to scribble a little greeting to you.
We've had our fun here at the hospital
Especially in room 210
Now you're heading home to Sandane
But I'm bound to see you again before too long
As you'll be back for outpatient's appointments.
I'm sure you'll be just as happy and up to your old
tricks.

Hug from Johanne

To Anne-Pia,

As a girl who's always good and kind
I will always bring you to mind
Full of joy with a real big smile
A lovely girl without any guile.

Lots of huge hugs from Torild.

Back in Oslo she writes in the blue diary that she's allowed to bathe in the bathtub, and that she's been into town with Aase and Margarethe, two adult girls from Sandane who live in Oslo. She goes to the cinema with Aase and Margarethe before they go for a meal at McDonald's and afterwards to the Theatre Café.

When Dad comes to collect her from the hospital, she comes rolling towards him with a smile. 'Dad, I've learned a joke. Do you want to hear it? There was a blind man, a bald man and a wheel-chair user who went to the Dead Sea because they'd heard that miracles could happen if you swam in it. The bald man went into the water first and came out with a beautiful head of hair. Then the blind man went into the water and when he came out he could see. Then the wheelchair user went into the water and when he came out he'd got new tyres on his chair!'

It's quite different on a plane when you're paralysed. Dad lifts her up onto his back to get her into the aircraft. Suddenly everything has become so much more bother.

I don't remember the first days after I came home. It's odd that I don't remember the moment when I became lame either. I do remember my time at Sophies Minde, but then it's blank again from the time I came home. Memory can be selective. Memory has probably understood and repressed the fact that it was more difficult to be at home in the new situation than it was in the hospital. I've been told that I wasn't always the easiest person to have around. But I don't actually remember anything of what it was like to be at home, whether anything changed between me and my brothers or sister or between my parents and me.

I have suppressed the memory of the first few months at home and yet the rehabilitation which followed is in the forefront of my memory. In April I was admitted to the Central Hospital in Førde (much nearer home) for a period of training me to 'function normally' again.

I wrote in the blue diary: *I am going to Førde . I am getting Dixie (Barbie's foal).*

The Central Hospital in Førde has a department for training people to do things which previously have come automatically, but which now have become a challenge several times a day. For example, putting your clothes on in bed can easily take half an hour. The occupational therapist stands beside my bed and makes helpful suggestions whilst entertaining me with a song:

Hum, hum, hum, hum;
I must run, run, run, run.
Dum, dum, dum, dum
Then I can come, come, come
In time for the last bus home.

Then there's the need to learn to get out of bed and into the wheelchair – and back again. She concentrates on finding good places to grip, lift her upper body with her arms and swing across the wheel. She has to watch that she doesn't lose her grip so that she loses her balance and ends up on the floor. Before she's able to do it properly she has a slide tray over the wheel between the chair and the bed. This tray makes it easier to slide across.

A wheelchair has to be adapted. It needs to be good to sit in, give support to the back, she needs to be able to roll along easily, turn corners and go backwards and forwards. Her legs need to rest securely on the footrest. The cushion must prevent pressure sores. There need to be handles at the back for pushing with. After having tried many and eventually found the right chair, she needs to get used to sitting in it, and get used to using it. That means that she needs to learn to manoeuvre the wheelchair without being afraid of falling backwards. The physiotherapist stands behind her when she puts her hands well back on the wheels, leans back and gets ready to tip the chair up onto its back wheels. The physiotherapist is behind and the support wheels are on. She knows this, but even so she's afraid of losing control. She needs to learn confidence that she will manage on her own and not be afraid. To turn the chair it's easier to turn the one wheel forwards at the same time as turning the other backwards.

I n the blue diary from the savings bank she writes:

Ingunn and I rode in the electric wheelchair <u>without permission</u>. If the occupational and physiotherapists had found out, I wouldn't have been allowed until I was bigger. A nurse (Turid) and I went to get some lilac plants from a man and saw horses at a stables on a farm.

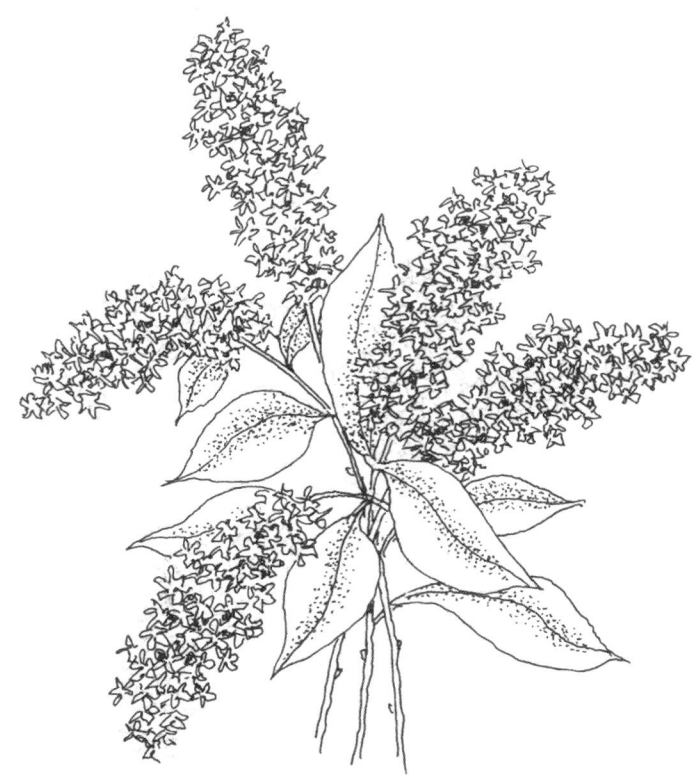

Following well-meaning advice she starts to drink a mixture of sour milk and vinegar. It makes a lumpy milk soup which smells nasty and uninviting, and tastes just as bad. Popular weekly magazines have made it into a fad, and a supposedly effective slimming food. It is for her own good.

I know full well because it's what they say: it's for my own good. It's always for my own good. I just wonder why I feel so against doing things for my own good. Why do I think I need to eat all kinds of other food than that which is good for me? Why do I buy chocolate which I gobble up without anybody seeing? Why I am I never full after a meal when other people only seem to play with their food?

THE HEALER

A healer comes to the ward just to meet her. They are sitting at a table in the communal kitchen and playing cards. When the unknown man comes in and sits himself down he holds his hand a couple of centimetres over her spine. He was expected that day, but even so his arrival seemed sudden. No introduction, just straight to the job. The healer gains the attention of everybody in the room, especially when, with his free hand, he magically produces a coin out of thin air.

After sitting a while at the kitchen table he asks whether he, and the lady who is with him, can continue treatment in her room. She lies on her bed and the healer sits beside her, holding his hands a few centimetres above her body.

'Can you feel the warmth?' he asks. She can't be completely sure, but yes, she does feel some warmth.

'You have a strong heart,' he says. 'I felt it straight away.'

She smiles. That, at least, was good news.

Now that she's only an hour and a quarter away from home, Mum and Dad come and collect her every weekend.

Mum has arranged with the leaders of the 4H club that she can have knitting as her activity. It's more practical than woodcarving. Since she can no longer just pop to the neighbours, Ragnhild has to come up to her, or they have to get some adults to help her up and down the steep hill between the houses.

One weekend, when Dad's going to collect her from the hospital, there's a certain amount of fuss before he comes. A rumour has gone round the mums in the ward that she's got a good-looking dad. 'When's your Dad coming to collect you?' ask the mums who are sitting in the dayroom, knitting. When he eventually arrives, everybody in the room falls silent. It's difficult to read Dad's body language to know whether he knows what's going on or not.

On the way home, Dad stops the car in Moskog and buys chicken for her. 'But don't tell your Mum,' he says. When he drives her back again on Sunday evening, he points out the red and white striped TV antenna, sitting regally on the top of Førde Mountain. In a strongly-convincing voice which can convey nothing but the truth, he says 'That there is where Eric Bye has his cabin.' Eric Bye is a Norwegian artist, author, film actor, folk singer and television celebrity. And Dad's hero. The family canoe is called Eric Bye.

When she gets back on the children's ward she hears that the mothers did in fact like what they saw. She doesn't really understand what all the fuss is about, but she tells Dad about it afterwards, anyway, even though she knows it will bolster his ego... And of course he is flattered and walks on cloud nine for a long time. And he doesn't easily let the family forget that there are people around who find him more exciting than they do. After she's been chatting with the mothers she goes out into the hallway to look at the mountain. Every time she looks up at the TV mast she thinks about her Dad and Eric Bye. And, somehow or other, it's good and safe to spend time thinking that the TV mast is Eric Bye's cabin.

HOSPITAL POEM

The hospital teacher, Kari, tells her to write a poem about the hospital. They do it together.

The occupational therapist helps all she can
She always finishes what she began
When we need help and advice
She's there in a trice.

The physiotherapist is dressed all in white
Britt who trains me day and night
Does just the same;
She really knows her game.
She will help me learn to stand
And anything else that comes to hand.

On the children's ward it's small people you find
The staff there are so very kind -
Apart from those with needles and pain
For they bring just misery and strain.
Whatever we play it's fun just the same
Doctors and nurses is the very best game.

Kari is taking her to a Jørn Hoel concert. Jørn Hoel is a singer, composer and solo artist; Runa, one of the nurses in the children's ward, is a lifelong Jørn Hoel fan. When she gets to hear about it she makes her promise to get his autograph. Runa cuts out a little piece of white paper and sticks it onto a bigger piece of red paper. 'That's where Jørn Hoel needs to sign,' says Runa and gives her the red piece of paper. Yet again she seriously promises that she'll manage it.

After the concert there's a queue backstage of people wanting to catch a glimpse of Jørn Hoel. When it's her turn she hands him Runa's home-made red note without a word, but then he asks her name. She wasn't expecting that. There's no way you can stand straight in front of Jørn Hoel and lie the first time you've ever met him. The only other autograph she's got is from the children's television character Big Bird, and he didn't need her name. She thought it was going to be easy-peasy to get the autograph for Runa and tried to explain to Jørn Hoel that she didn't want it for herself.

'Is it a little girl like you who's going to have it?', he asks. She realises she's wasting time. 'Yes', she replies. What else could she say? The only other possible answer was 'No, it's for an adult and I don't know how old she is, but she's grown up and works on the children's ward where I am, but she's been so artistic in making this card and she thinks you're great and please sign it because I've promised her' – and surely it doesn't matter that she's not a little girl like me? 'Yes, she's a little girl just like me'. He writes, *Loveliest wishes to Runa.*

And then he asks whether she doesn't want his autograph as well. She's a bit confused because she actually hadn't thought about that at all and she hasn't got any more paper. She turns round, but the people behind her, waiting for his autograph, have only got enough paper for their own use.

So she turns back to Jørn Hoel and shakes her head.

The class are coming to the hospital on a visit. They're allowed into the physiotherapy room, where she has her training sessions, and into the schoolroom.

Kari wants her to play the synthesiser for the class – something she's reluctant to do. By means of a bit of cheating, Kari manages to convince her. Before the class arrives, they plan that she's going to turn on one of the pre-recorded background rhythms on the synthesiser and then act as though it's her that's playing. In that way she'll be able to impress the class without being afraid of hitting wrong notes. Nevertheless she's nervous. And because she's so nervous, when she 'plays' for the class it's difficult to watch their faces to see whether anybody realises she's cheating. She chooses to focus her attention on the synthesiser and watches her fingers on the notes the whole time.

When the song's finished one of the teachers, who is on the trip and actually teaches music, is thrilled. 'Gosh! You're so clever,' she says admiringly, clapping her hands together.

The class are going on to the swimming pool in Førde, and when they've gone she and Kari can at last fall about laughing at their well-played joke. She's surprised at herself. Just think that she managed it! She looks up to Kari, who is the best and most fun teacher that the hospital has ever had.

SALE OF SALT-DOUGH FIGURES AND PICTURES

One of the bed-bound children in the children's ward is often visited by her parents and her sister, Monica. She gets to know Monica and one day they decide they're going to raise money for a good cause. They draw pictures and make salt-dough characters, and then go round the different wards selling what they've made. Ingunn helps them find a good cause and suggests that they open a fund in the name of a child who had died of cancer at the hospital. The response is very good. They manage to sell everything they've made, and make 200 kroner.

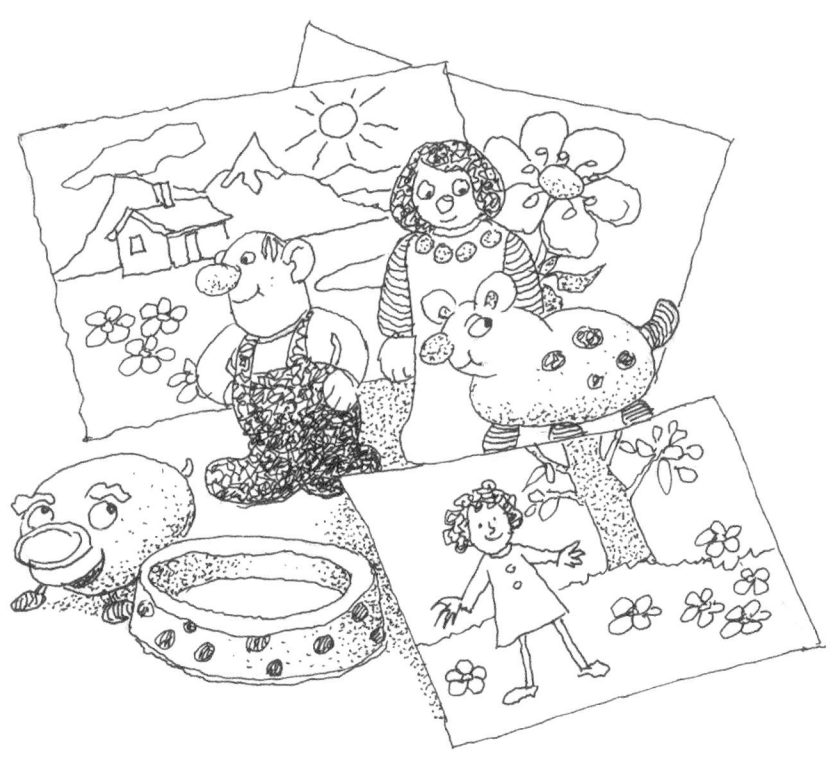

In the blue diary it says:

Went to Sophies Minde as an outpatient but ended up being admitted.

A short poem scribbled there:

No-one can see that I'm dancing
No-one can see that I run
No-one can see that I'm jumping
No-one can see that I walk.
No-one can see that I wiggle my big toe
Or that I react when I'm tickled.
But everyone sees that I sit in my wheelchair
But you'd better have eyes like a hawk
Because very soon I'll walk.

19 September

Travel to Sunnaas for training. Inger Johanne comes too.

She's eleven years old on her first stay at Sunnaas. Her eleventh birthday was celebrated in Førde Central Hospital with Grandma, Grandpa and Ranghild as guests.

The other patients at Sunnaas are adults, but quite nice, and on every visit she gets her horizons widened. She gets to hear about diving accidents, climbing accidents and car accidents. All of them were once young and full of life, and they're not totally lifeless now, even though life now is totally different for those who end up in room 6.

Room 6 at Sunnaas is the ward where those who have been involved in road traffic accidents and those who have had spinal surgery come to recuperate and prepare for a new life-situation. Here, there's far more laughter than you'd expect with so many seriously-injured people together. Lots of those who work here help keep the merry atmosphere going, but it's not the same as at Sophies Minde.

I was in the mat group today. That means that I had to roll around on the mats, throw a ball and do press-ups. I did archery as well. Vivian has made a timetable for me today. Tomorrow I'm going to the swimming pool, playing volleyball and going to the occupational therapist.

She and a young lad are the youngest there that first time. She's two years younger and, compared to him, she feels clumsy and awkward since she doesn't manage to crawl at full speed across the floor and then swish up into her wheelchair again. Those who are a bit older are well trained and joke with each other about everything. The young adults and teenagers in wheelchairs sit together in the dayroom, smoking and laughing.

The other patients are nice, it's not that they're not, but all these impressions are overwhelming for a shy eleven-year-old from Western Norway, and so it ends up with me sitting alone in my room because I don't dare go into the television room in case someone else is there. Again I feel very small, clumsy, vulnerable and very, very lonely. The people who work at Sunnaas are very kind, but they haven't got time to talk to me so I end up sitting alone in my room.

At Sunnaas she's been offered an appointment with a psychiatrist. A lady comes to her room and introduces herself.

'Is there anything you want to talk about?' asks the psychiatrist.

But she doesn't manage to find anything to talk about.

'How are you?' asks the psychiatrist.

She replies, 'all right,' the same as she always does to that question. It's an automatic response. It's become a habit always to answer positively, whatever the question is. Everything is less complicated if she says that it's fine, so that's what she says. She says that she's fine.

The truth is that things are fine during the day. It's in the evening the thoughts come and things aren't so easy any longer. But that's the way it's been as long as I can remember. I hardly know anything else. The painful thoughts have become such a natural part of me, that even when these thoughts come during the day I've started to think that's the way it's meant to be. It's nothing to reflect over, there's nothing anyone can do about it. Nor has anyone talked about it being natural to be like this, so I think it must just be my problem. The dark days just make me appreciate all the more the good times I have with people. When I get letters from home or when the nurses come into my room to measure my temperature or give me tablets, or when I can play in peace with my Barbie dolls.

Then the psychiatrist asks about my family. But everything's fine there too. She's got nothing left to say, nothing to ask about. No feelings she can just put her finger on. There was no dramatic car journey which turned life upside down, no violence, no sudden happening. When she was paralysed it happened gradually and slowly. So slowly now that, even such a short time afterwards, she seems to have accepted the situation. She can't compete with the other patients' fates, so what's she meant to talk to the psychiatrist about?

And also, just now she is alright because Dad's outside waiting for her, and she knows he's going home soon. She wants to spend her time on him, not on the psychiatrist. The psychiatrist doesn't get anything else out of her and concludes that she's fine. They say goodbye and don't see one another again.

BACK TO CLASS

When she gets to move back home after months away, she's been gone so long that she doesn't know the people whom her classmates are talking about. Things that they've taken part in, both in school and out of school, she's missed out on. As well as that, she's now in a wheelchair. For the first four years of her schooling she's been to and fro from hospital, and still looks like the rest of them, so managed to re-connect with life at home. This time it's all different. She knows everything about her body and what's wrong with her, and why it's happened.

She's told her story so many different times to so many different people. It's all so familiar, the doors and the corners at Sophies Minde and Sunnaas, the feel of the walls when you touch them, and she can at any time recall the smell of perfume and cigarettes from the staff room at Sophies. She knows how a doctor studies an X-ray picture and then comes up to you to press your stomach and back, how cold she can feel and just wants to put on a jumper again. She can talk about how long it takes to get dressed in bed, and how it's even longer when you're sitting on a shower chair. She can try to explain why everything would have been so much easier if only she'd had Mum and Dad with her the whole time, but she'll never talk about all the nights when she's lain awake crying because she feels so lonely, or because she feels so inferior to all the others. The footrest, the wheels on her wheelchair and how they affect the tipping point, the slide board, shower and toilet stool, catheters and wee bags, leg splints, cutlery with handles, electronic kitchen work surfaces, electric wheelchairs, stretch-fitted sheets, nappies, bed hoists, injections, arm exercises, leg exercises, practical trousers, practical colours, her own diet, healthy food and unhealthy food, dietary advice from the kitchen, wheeling the chair outside, maintenance of the chair, practicing going up kerbs, toilet training, nurses, physiotherapists, occupational therapists, long corridors. She knows lots about these and many other things, but she doesn't think her classmates would be very interested.

They talk about other boys and girls, collecting things, sports and fashion. A world that she hasn't been a part of. And that's why she sticks out. They see it in the wheelchair that she has become another person.

What sort of person was I that day? An alien? No. Not even that. A stone. I'd become a stone that just was there.

Nobody wants to be with her. The craze at the moment for girls is skipping and Chinese elastic (French skipping or jump rope). She holds one end of the rope when they skip. It's boring and she doesn't really want to, but it's the only way she can join in. Otherwise she just has to sit and watch. French skipping she can't join in with at all.

At the class party she's pleased when one of the boys wants to dance with her, even though dancing only means holding other others' hands and swinging backwards and forwards. At the end of the dance she discovers it was the girls in the class who asked him to dance with her. She realises that they mean well, but none of the boys need forcing to ask any of the other girls to dance. She's embarrassed and feels in the way for the rest of the evening. Everything has changed in relation to her classmates. She can feel the distance between herself and them.

Of course, I'm not very interesting. I can't do what the others can do. I can't go where the others go. I wasn't here when the boys, without getting caught, sneaked behind the school to have a smoke. I realise I'm missing out when the boys chase the girls with a dead mouse, but don't ever come near me.

It is as if she has been divided in two.

One who is healthy, who thinks like well people, dreams about what she will be when she grows up and can do everything well people can do.

At the same time she is someone who is unwell, someone who can't spend time thinking about the future because she has to concentrate on finding out how to cope with using a wheelchair, how her room should be, her house and school. How to get outside to join in or watch all the things healthy children do.

Many people can only see her as disabled, few see the healthy individual. She sees herself as healthy, despite using a wheelchair. But there are circumstances that mean she begins to see herself as disabled and unwell. It is confusing to work out which of the two identities she is.

Janne

Janne is her second cousin; she is in the class below her. Janne would do anything if it means that she would be able to walk again. Would even give away her toys. It is only when they have playtime at the same time that she has someone who actually wants to be with her. She still feels like herself when she is with Janne.

A doctor comes to visit the class to explain what has happened to her. '…And it could be that she might have an "accident" but you mustn't think it is her fault. She can't feel when she needs to go to the toilet.'

She wishes the floor would swallow her up. She thinks, *beam me up, Scotty*! If that is what the doctor came to say then she thinks he should never have come. She has a nasty suspicion that this information talk will not improve her relationship with the others one bit! This will make it even more difficult for them to see her has normal.

She just sits there

It does not appear that her teachers have had any information about how to relate to her either. They don't let her join in with the others at all.

Even if it was only helping to tidy away the books, she would have felt that she was of some use, allowed to be one of them, to complain about how boring it is tidying books, laugh about something they find in a box in the cellar.

She sits there as the others go back and forth.

She doesn't know what to do, so she just sits there.

She doesn't know what to say so, she just sits there.

At playtime Hildegunn pushes her into the wall of a shelter. She does not mean to. They are having a piggy-back race in pairs. Hildegunn holds the handles at the back of her chair and runs.

On the way back Hildegunn lets go of the wheelchair a bit too soon. The chair carries on rolling at speed. Secure in the misplaced trust that Hildegunn is still in control of the chair she sits back with her hands in her lap. Into the wall with a hard fast thump. Luckily her nose takes the worst of the bump and she soon recovers without any lasting damage. Her nose throbs, though. Hildegunn has a much worse time of it, despite her assurances that she is fine; she knows it was an accident and not intentional, there is no harm done. The following day Hildegunn brings her a present as she feels so bad about the accident.

Another time she falls out of her wheelchair right at the head teacher's feet! Dratted doorsteps!

But I wish it happened more often, both of these events, because it means I can laugh at myself with the others.

The only place she can express her hopes and dreams is when she plays by herself. It is therapeutic. She allows herself to be overwhelmed by her innermost thoughts, the ones she feels she cannot say to anyone. Inside she is still the same but not many people realise it.

New furniture.
Instead of a settee bed, hospital bed.
Instead of an office chair, wheelchair.
And then her room is full.

Suddenly my room is no longer as it was.
Suddenly I am no longer as I was.

Eventually the room has to be extended as it is too small and too impractical. The occupational therapist comes with inspiration and good advice. *Having it that way is the most practical. We need to find a better solution for that.* Out with the old and in with the new. Everything will be so good. So very practical, not at all as it was before.

Why am I not enthusiastic, get involved in the way I ought? Listen to what they say, smile and nod, agree, agree. All the practical stuff doesn't interest me. It is nothing to do with me. I am empty inside. Anything that bubbles up I press down again until it is gone.

It seems that everyone has forgotten who I am and that confuses me. I am adaptable. I will soon manage to forget who I am. I know that people looked at me strangely before too. I know that I wasn't like all the others, I could see that in the mirror. I was however Anne-Pia. Now… now there are fewer things I can join in with and that matters to others. Is that what they think at school; she can't help, she can't join in the games any longer, it is best to stay away from her?

How can I say that I am still me when I am not sure myself who I am? How can I help them understand when I don't understand any more? I don't want to go to school, I don't want to be happy, I don't want to be me any more. I want to be a better version of myself, someone others can like. Not this. Soon, hopefully, I will manage to forget who I am and all that I could have been.

Things improve a little the following year. Her experiences on her last visit have come out, and so now some of the nurses spend a bit more time with her. She can go out in the evenings, go home with some of them and get to know their families.

When she and Dad travel to Sunnaas they have to get up at 5 a.m. to make the flight which goes at 7 a.m. They land first at Sogndal where passengers for Bergen change planes, then at Oslo. From the airport they take a taxi to the quayside, a boat to Nesoddtangen and then a bus to Sunnaas.

We arrive at Sunnaas at about 9.30 a.m. At Sunnaas we see a doctor and some others. Dad has to head home at 3.15 p.m. It is sad but at 3.30 there is archery and I am doing it, so I completely forget to be sad. At 4 p.m. I have lobscouse and crackers for dinner. From 5-7 p.m. there is table tennis so there is a lot to do before I fall asleep at about 10.02 p.m.

Room 6 at Sunnaas is a training ward where those with spinal injuries recuperate and learn the physical skills necessary for their new life. This is a tough process that can take many months. It is not only about physical strength; you have to re-learn basic skills, too. You have to learn to be as independent as possible in all regular activities. There is also social training, something she feels she lacks. Without knowing how others see her, she thinks of herself as a girl who smiles but then withdraws, only to blame herself afterwards for not being brave enough to dare to have views, to dare to be a nuisance.

The summer she is thirteen she gets to know Katrine, who is two years younger and is completely paralysed after a road accident between a car and horse. She is glad to have someone she dares to spend time with, someone to talk to. They are taken to Tusenfryd fairground theatre where they see a show.

On the way out of Tusenfryd she is left at the top of an escalator, the one you have to use to get from the entrance to the fairground. The nurses are helping other wheelchair users down and she is waiting for her turn. Then the fairground director Aase Kleveland comes and wants to help. At last it is her turn and, with her back to the steps, a nurse behind and Aase Kleveland at the front, they begin their descent.

When they get to the bottom there is a bit of confusion and jockeying for position. Aase Kleveland has to step over her to get to the other side. Aase Kleveland lifts her foot up and her knee hits her in the forehead. She shakes her head gently while Aase Kleveland apologises and asks how she is. She smiles politely, 'I'm fine.'

In her new bedroom she has a telephone socket and her own telephone provided by the technical aids' office. Ragnhild is in the new room with her. It is almost like before. She can be her real self, the healthy self, when she is with Ragnhild.

They ring the chat line and use false names when talking to the others who have also rung the chat line. They usually claim to be older than they really are. Age has become more important since an operator has been employed to remove users who are under eighteen. If the operator suspects that a user is under eighteen she can interrupt the conversation and ask certain questions. If you are discovered you are asked to hang up. It is best to make a list in advance of answers to any such questions including age, date of birth, which year you left Year 9 at secondary school, and other things the operator might ask.

It's Ragnhild who first speaks to speaks to Joakim. After chatting away for a while she suddenly says, 'My friend is in a wheelchair too, just a minute and you can speak to her!' She passes the phone over and Joakim is on the other end.

Later, during the summer holidays at Sunnaas, she meets Joakim face to face! When she realises it's him she has spoken to on the phone she is embarrassed and wishes the floor would swallow her up. But then Joakim also makes the connection. When he too realises they have spoken before, their conversation becomes more natural and suddenly it is all alright – she is no longer embarrassed.

Another time when they ring the chat line she gets into a conversation with a man who wants to ring her privately. She has of course given a false name and she makes up a false phone number. She and Ragnhild giggle about what he will say when he rings the false number and asks after Karin, and Karin doesn't live there. The phone number is written in her school diary under 'secret'.

Most patients in room 6 are in their twenties. They are slim and seem to manage everything they work towards.

The sneaking suspicion comes more and more often here at Sunnaas. That it is not only with able-bodied people that she doesn't quite fit in.

Here she comes, little and round, out for a roll around the hospital with them. From several feet behind she sees that they manoeuvre their wheelchairs as if they are no hindrance while she has already had enough after the first corner! She sees them chat and laugh with the physiotherapists walking along beside them, while she has barely enough breath to focus on her wheelchair driving. Then they stop to practice their wheelchair safety. The do things like jumping up a small curb, balancing on their back wheels, go down a curb on their back wheels, before going in to practice falling backwards in a wheelchair, using their hands to recover themselves and pushing up the same way.

The popular way to get from floor to chair is to place one hand on the floor, the other hand on the chair then quite simply lift yourself up. It looks simple when someone does it and it seems to her that everyone can do it, except her. There are other ways to do it, though. She sits on the floor in front of the chair. The physiotherapist stands behind her. 'You can do it, come on!' Yet again she positions one foot behind the other, twists her upper body and gets ready. Then she is on her knees whilst hanging on to the wheelchair to support herself. 'That's it! I will grab your trousers and on the count of three lift yourself up with your arms, twist round, and you will be sitting in your chair!' One, two, three, she pushes with her arms and twists. When she looks around she hasn't moved an inch, but her arms are tired and she sinks down into a heap on the floor. 'Have a little break then we'll try again!'

Mat work with the same group is another challenge. Balancing on their knees, they are to hold on tightly to the huge ball in the middle of the mat. You have to pull the ball towards yourself and cause all the others to lose their balance and drop like flies onto the mat (this is not too difficult when you are against people who are paralysed over a large portion of their body).

The first problem is getting into the start position. This involves pulling your body up and towards the ball then staying there until the game begins. She is the first to fall, with a slow groan. As soon as the ball begins to move, she falls off her knees.

Aunt Grete comes to take her home to Holmlia. She only goes for training in the summer, so she is not at Holmlia every weekend as she had been in the past.

She has written a short poem and stories in her diary. When she tells her aunt and the others about it they convince her to read them aloud after dinner.

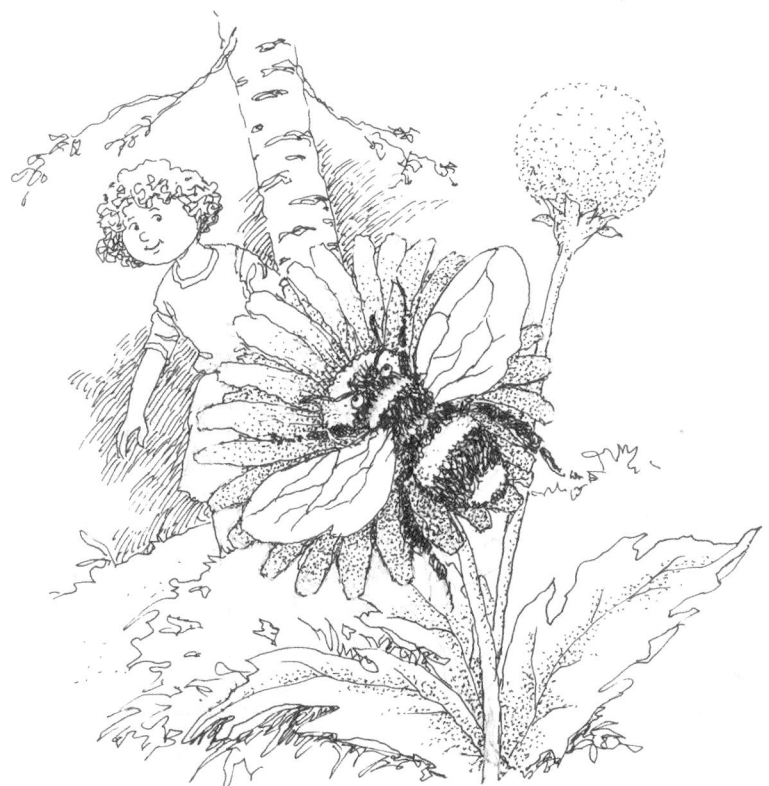

The flower drama!!

Round and round buzz the bees,
There's a flower in between some trees.
The bees want their honey but here comes a girl so sunny!
She sees the flower and thinks it's fair,
She smells it but the bees are already there!!
Suddenly she jumps up in surprise; the bees have stung her between the eyes.
The bees think she is rather wet; but don't stop long: there's honey to get.

Since Janne lives far out in the country, every visit has to be planned at school the day before, or over the phone. They dream of being famous, and get a foretaste of such fame at the school end-of-year show. They perform for the whole secondary school. They have written the text themselves and the music is Let it swing. First they have to ask the Head for permission to perform. When he is happy with their proposal they ask him to keep it a secret. Nobody else is to know about their performance in advance. It will be a surprise. The only other person who needs to know is the music teacher who will accompany them on the piano. They have to practice together. They go to the music teacher's home.

The big evening arrives. The end of her time in secondary school; she has been looking forward to this. Looking forward to a new start somewhere else. A clean sheet! Recently things have been difficult, not bright and cheerful. It is fitting to finish on this note. A reminder that she will be herself, the person almost nobody thinks she can be. Even in her wheelchair she is half of Bobby Socks or The Japps, which is what they call themselves as they sit in front of the cassette player and sing songs they have written themselves. Janne, Anne-Pia, Peter, Stian. JAPPS. Their brothers didn't often perform as backing singers even though they got their initials in the band name.

Before the performance they put on their make up so as to be ready when their turn comes. She likes to be a girly-girl. She can remember three or four Christmases ago getting a present with clip-on ear rings, ring, bracelet, necklace. There was even lipstick, eye shadow, mascara and rouge in it. On top of all that there was also a silver tiara with a big blue stone (of plastic) in the middle surrounded by small round stones in the same colour. She felt beautiful. Mum said she was beautiful. Paul and Peter said she looked girly. She dreamt of being a princess so she could wear ball gowns, make-up and jewellery every day, or perhaps a ballerina with a tutu, pale-pink ballet shoes and white, nearly-see-through tights.

When they come out of the dressing room they bow their heads so nobody can see that they have make-up on; nobody knows yet that they are going on stage to sing. The make-up feels heavy; it doesn't make her feel good. She knows that nobody expects her to look good. It feels odd to be on stage. The butterflies flutter right through her body as she looks out into the gym hall.

One Friday while we were in town
We heard music coming from a disco
And decided that we wanted to
Come in and hear more
And more…

She sees the surprised faces and at the end of the song the audience begins to clap in time to the final chorus. This is how being famous feels; being on stage and looking out towards a smiling audience, who like what you do. It was such a surprise for them. This makes her feel good, feel good and be seen. If only this moment could last for ever!

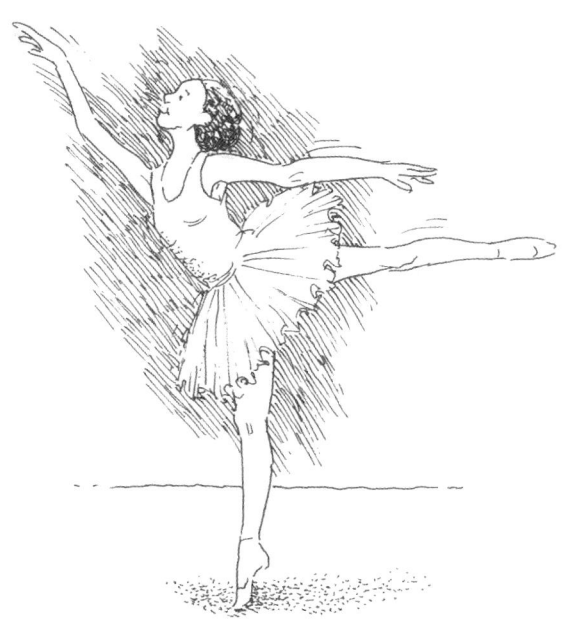

FIRST VISIT TO BEITOSTØLEN HEALTH SPORTS CENTRE

Monday 23 March 1990

We arrived at Beitostølen health sports centre at 4:30 p.m. (approx). The bus ride had taken roughly seven hours. We spoke to a nurse on arrival. It was a man. We were shown round. It is a nice building but I think it resembles a hospital!

Tuesday

Una and I each speak to our doctor. The one I spoke to was Danish. Activities don't begin until tomorrow, I am told. We also met the physiotherapist. She has worked at Sunnaas. There are horses and dogs here. We are invited into the stables. They have birds there too. The evening was spent in the hotel, which had a theme evening about the Valdres area in southern Norway.

Wednesday

We swam today. It was wonderful. Afterwards it was time for school: I did maths. After that, Svein and I went to the fitness room. We had hard training. I drove a dog sleigh, which was cool! In the evening we went to the gym. Almost everyone took part in the 'health dance'. It was somewhat strange but otherwise OK!

Thursday

Swimming today too! The water was a bit cooler than yesterday. Afterwards we went horse riding. The saddle had a handle for me to hold. The horse was a Dølehest or Dole horse and called Sandra. We made Easter decorations. Mum rang. I got to bed at about 10.30 p.m.!

Friday

The staff entertained us during the evening. It was great!! This was followed by a dance. I joined in. It is better dancing here than at home. I think this is because people dare to dance with wheelchair users here. They are perhaps less shy. Perhaps someone thinks, 'Oh, she can't dance because of her wheelchair, can she?' I think that's stupid. I wish I was as good at wheelchair dancing as the people we see on TV!

Sunday

Today is April Fool's Day. I have fooled Una and Svein with, 'Look, there's someone over there!' and, 'look, what's that, isn't it a tiny bird/squirrel?'

Or I point at something and stare at it petrified. The others wonder what it is and look in the direction I'm pointing. Then I say, 'April fool!' really quickly.

Tuesday

After riding I had to go down to the cellar room to work out with weights, and to practice getting into my wheelchair from the floor. I think if it is so difficult to get back in my chair I would rather stay on the floor!

P.S. There was a boy last week who recognised my name. He said we had been at Sophies Minde together some years ago. He plays the accordion very well!

Thursday

We have been out sledging today. It was wild! When I went down I was going at least sixty miles per hour and it is just typical that I have to find the only jump on the hill. I went at least ten feet in the air. Amazingly I didn't fall off. I had three goes. If you are wondering how I got back up the hill, Magnar took the sledge rope around his waist and dragged me up.

Since she is now regularly at the health sports centre she discovers that she has had far too much help wheeling her chair. Even if they are in a rush, and the roads are stony, it is more satisfying for her to get herself to and from places. She sees it in the others who manage alone and realises that it is silly to have too much help when she can manage alone with a bit of training.

When she comes home she practices wheeling her chair bit by bit while they are out. When Mum and Dad automatically begin to push her chair she grabs the wheels and would rather do it herself. It is difficult to take away Mum and Dad's responsibility because she knows that they are only trying to help, but there are so many other things she still needs their help with. In the end, without anything being said, they understand that there are some things that she wants to do herself and that she will ask when she is really stuck and needs help.

To begin with, the skin on her hands becomes hard and full of dirt and sores. At Beitostølen she is told about good hand cream and gloves.

Another thing she learns there is that she is not alone. There are other people just like her, although they are very different individuals. They have the same thoughts she has, the thoughts that nobody at home knows about.

When she comes home after a summer at Beitostølen she has a new vigour. Energy that has come from her new friends. All of these young men and women are so much more than they are able to show at home. At Beitostølen the wheelchairs, crutches or those invisible things that no-one is aware of but nevertheless mean that people look at you funnily, mean absolutely nothing. The helpers and instructors are young men and women who know that she is more than just a girl in a wheelchair. For a month, every other summer, she is with others who know and understand.

They give her normal things to chat about with her friends at home. These are the usual things to be interested in: pubs, Peppes Pizza, outings to mountain lakes, barbeques, shopping in Fagernes city, boys, music, people, discos in the school gym hall, swimming, air-rifle shooting, darts, painting your own pictures on t-shirts or making your own belts and jewellery.

She meets people from other parts of the country at Beitostølen. They live a long way from her. Her own county has a very scattered population, and she is the only person in her village with paralysed legs. A short time after she started to use her wheelchair her parents were contacted by the Association for Handicapped Children's Parents who encouraged them to join the Norwegian Handicap Association. The family starts to go to events arranged by the Association for Handicapped Children's Parents in her home county. She meets children with different handicaps. It was great in the beginning, fun to get to know new people, but before long the events remind her of something she is trying to escape from. The fact that she is handicapped, different from the others at home.

These gatherings are unlike Beitostølen because participants are more dependent on their parents and the organised activities such as orienteering and boccia (An internationally-played sport developed particularly for wheelchair users. It is similar to bowls although balls are thrown rather than rolled.) They are not necessarily the things she would want to do. There is nothing interesting there to chat with her class mates about. She doesn't want her new friends to connect her with illness, difference or with being dependent on help.

She knows they go to these events for her sake, but it doesn't feel that way. She doesn't want to be compared with disabled people. She doesn't want to be disabled, doesn't want to have anything in common with them; why does nobody see that?! Why is she forced to go there?!

She had never imagined that life would be like this. She had been promised that everything would be OK again. It even said so in a national magazine:

Now that the treatment is finished Anne-Pia can hopefully look forward to a future with the same expectations as most other people.

The last thing she had thought was that she would have a future that was about illness, abnormality, being different. That chapter was supposed to be closed. Bit by bit she gets used to being dependant on her wheelchair. It feels good no longer to have to balance on painful weak legs. If she can practice enough wheelchair driving technique she can be a normal girl. For a moment she thinks that the only difference is in not being able to walk. It isn't until she is in her mid-teens that she realises the full consequences of the medical mistakes. Like small insect bites the changes have been there all along but she had managed to deny that they mattered.

A bite when, from her bedroom window, she hears two of her friends walking down the road happy and laughing on their way to or from something.

A bite when, on a school trip, she had to be so dependent on help from an adult that it was difficult to feel like one of the class.

A bite when she has to ask for help to pee after dinner when Mum and Dad usually relax. She feels like she is a nuisance to them.

Frustration because her body has let her down and she cannot join in the activities she was a part of before. She has had music lessons on the organ, has just started to play the fiddle, but had to stop because it was too difficult to stand. Holding the fiddle was too difficult for her back. Then she was paralysed and had to stop everything. They had to find alternative activities for her. That is how she came to start playing the synthesiser. Her music teacher lets her play drums, or jam blues on the piano when the synth gets boring. She is allowed because he realises that she will never be an expert anyway. She has not got piano fingers. She can't manage the simplest chords with her left hand. It is more fun to play freely on the drums or play the blues.

Her care assistant takes her out to do things together, to socialise with her. She knows the drill and has fun with what turns out to be three care assistants. It is a bit like having a big sister and yet not because they are called care assistants. She has to refer to them as care assistants when she is explaining whom she has been out with to Ragnhild and Janne. Others don't have need of such support, just those who have something wrong with them.

She goes to the archery club and plays the synth at music lessons. But besides these organised activities she's much on her own. And because she is so often alone, her imagination explodes into a private kingdom in which she rules. All the wonder and passion she can imagine is lived out in the world of the written word – both her own and others' – and her Barbie dolls are the only ones she shares this with. She lets them live the life she lives in her thoughts.

At the same time she spins dreams that even dolls aren't allowed to be part of. A secret wish to experience one day the life and passion she reads about. Passionate love, and that someone would be able to love her just as much in return. Passion for a job, such as an artist with her own studio, trips abroad and exhibitions, surrounded by wonderful clothes and tall champagne glasses. Her in the centre. That such a life can still be for her in the future, despite the voice inside her becoming louder and louder. *You're not like the others. Your dreams don't matter any more. The others have moved on in life and you've ground to a halt.* She comforts herself in her private kingdom with its glittering treasures hidden in an Aladdin's cave.

She gets to know Inghild in the summer before she goes on to further education. They meet in a period where they're both vulnerable and struggling to find their place with others. Each of them feels out of it and although they each end up in parallel classes with a different circle of friends, Inghild comes and takes her out when she'd rather stay at home because home is a safe place.

As well as friendship with Inghild, she gets lots of new classmates and friends who see her for who she is. It's like entering another world. When she was in secondary school she never wanted to go; she would feel ill and didn't like it once she became dependent on her wheelchair. Now it doesn't take many days before she's actually part of a group that includes her in a very natural way. This strengthens her.

The District Nurse

A shadow which casts itself across everything is that she still needs help to pee, including at school. And because this is so embarrassing she tells her friends that the district nurse comes at lunchtime to help her strengthen her legs in the room which has been made for her. The room, which is locked and contains a bench, washing and toilet equipment, also becomes a training room with boring training sessions when she talks about it.

She's petrified that what she's actually doing in there will be discovered. Afraid of what the others will think of someone who needs help to go to the toilet. Afraid that they'll stop liking her and that she'll suddenly be without friends. Toilet matters are embarrassingly unpleasant for teenagers. 'That won't happen. They will understand', says the district nurse. 'You'll feel much better if you were honest about it, and you wouldn't have to lie any more'. She chooses not to believe that advice.

The summer after she finishes in Year 8 at secondary school, she goes to Sunnaas and Inghild comes to visit. They steal a cigarette and a match from a nurse and hide behind the hospital. She's not sure that she inhales the smoke properly. Lots of chewing gum and perfume before they put the box of matches back without being discovered.

After the holidays, when school begins again, they lock themselves in the toilets to have a smoke. They are discovered and she is told that she has to follow the same rules as everybody else despite being in a wheelchair. They giggle about it afterwards. Sometimes they don't go to the lessons. They sit in the toilets and chat. At home there are arguments with her parents because she is friends with someone who smokes, drinks and goes out in the evenings.

They only see what's wrong. They don't understand. It took me some time to see past the insecurity behind these actions. Insecurity, because it wasn't my usual style. Before I managed to discover what this experience would give me. Now I know that I need it. I need to be out amongst people. All sorts of people. It feels good to belong to different groups, both safe groups and less safe groups. It helps to make me normal. To help me socialise. Even though it will make it more obvious that I am different. But I'm able to show who I am and explore different situations. And when it all boils down to it, that's the most important.

They want to go to Oslo to a Guns 'n' Roses concert. Mum and Dad take some convincing.

'But you're only fifteen!'

'I'm never allowed to do anything. Please!'

After tears, shouting and promising they eventually get to Valle Hovin, the outdoor concert arena, along with lots of others. After several hours of waiting – first waiting to get into the arena, and then waiting through the warm-up band – at last, an hour and a half late, Guns n Roses are on stage. The terrace is way too far back but it is slightly raised so that they can see over the heads of the rest of the public. If it hadn't been for the huge screens it could have been anybody running up and down the stage; one with a top hat and black curly hair, and one with long red hair, tight boxer shorts and a T-shirt with a picture of Jesus. It would have been a good idea to bring binoculars. But the thrill of the music and the experience of being there gets to them and moves them deep inside. Only once the concert is over does she realise that her shoulders are sunburned.

They've had a good time, something she really appreciates because she and Inghild think and react differently, which is not always a good thing. But every time things settle down between them they are again full of song and laughter. Like when they're on the back seat of the car and she suddenly sees a local artist right outside the window. She points and shouts so that Inghild will see him. Inghild turns her head towards the window and then looks down at her. 'Oh, so, you do reach the window then,' says Inghild, appearing to be surprised and then giggling.

Back in her room she sits quietly and listens to Inghild talking about boys. She says as little as possible when they're on this subject because she doesn't feel she has anything to contribute. The same thoughts that she hears from others, appear within herself. But all the same, it feels as though boys are something reserved for everybody except her. Therefore she doesn't permit herself to speak openly about her thoughts. What is the worst thing that can happen? To be laughed at because she has those sorts of dreams for herself, or to be rejected by a boy and know that somebody thinks it's a shame for her because she has such hopes.

Camping at the little lake. It's really a big lake, surrounded by high mountains. Playful fish. No other tents or people in sight. Practically, it's an absolutely dreadful trip. It's the first and last time she stays in a tent. It rains, and the only positive aspect of that is that a morning dip in the lake is warm. Apart from that, personal hygiene isn't up to much. Ants in a piece of left-over cake, an unpleasant damp smell in the tent. But it's here that they talk about the future. Promise to be head bridesmaid for each other. She doesn't say it out loud but assumes that she will be head bridesmaid for Inghild but not the other way round.

At night in the town centre drunks stop for a chat. Often about the time they broke their foot and had to use a wheelchair. Or about more serious things that people they know have been through, in a difficult period. There are, as well, some people who feel that they have permission to ask about the most personal, private things and to expect an answer. It is flattering and irritating at the same time. People initiate contact because of the wheelchair: the exact thing she wants people to forget.

Situations that make it difficult outdoors.

Such as:
* How much can one drink without wanting to go to the toilet, and
* Where can I go to the toilet?
* How do I get home when I can't get into a telephone box to ring for a taxi and I suddenly appear to be the only person left in town?
* They got me up that steep stairwell but how will I get down again when everyone's asleep?
* Handicapped toilets used as storerooms.

At the Blakken club, the smoking corner in the billiard room is where everyone congregates. It's easy to talk to people here. It's perhaps to do with the fact that everyone sits, busy with their cigarette between their fingers, whilst giggling at a sticker that says 'kissing a smoker is like kissing an ashtray.'

On the dance floor with her friends she can really let her hair down. They dance alone and yet together in a ring. Everybody wiggles and wafts their arms and everything else that they can waft, and join in the lyrics. *What is love? Baby don't hurt me; don't hurt me anymore!*

In the winter it's cold out in the evenings. Everything's closed. She's in the town centre and has to ask somebody to ring from the phone box that she can't get into. She has to wait for a vacant taxi to come and get her. She gets home. They've forgotten to leave the door on the latch. She doesn't want to ring the doorbell because her little sisters are in bed, asleep. Mum's on an early shift tomorrow. She doesn't want to wake any of them. The hall is unlocked so she might as well sleep sitting in her wheelchair in the hall until Mum comes.

She uses her scooter-like electric wheelchair to get into town when they aren't being driven by Mum or Dad. It is this one that got a flat battery just before the last hill up to her house, and Linda had to run up and get Dad to come round the other way in the car.

One night out on the town a big bear of a chap who has had one too many comes to show off a bit. He suddenly jumps up on the front of the chair and it tips forward. She dangles there in the air, at a sixty-degree angle, for a few seconds before her friends come rushing over and push him away.

The scooter has three wheels and isn't very stable. This was the one she was allowed to apply for, because if she had been offered a four wheel model, which is more comfortable to sit in, the powers-that-be were afraid that she would want to use it all the time and so become lazy. It ended up being the scooter. If she hits a bump in the road without noticing it in time, the whole thing tips and she falls sideways out of it and into the road. The person behind with the manual wheelchair that she needs in order to be able to get indoors, tips too, but quickly jumps up to stop the traffic which is coming towards them.

She tried to go out in the garden with the scooter. The garden is big and on a hillside. She wants to go out there alone since the last time she was able to was when she could walk. She thought that the scooter was a good idea and would enable her to get across the grass. When she had managed to turn, and was on her way back again, she drove into a big stone hidden in the grass and tipped. Everything moved in slow motion. She could see Paul and Dad on the veranda, watching what happened. She was not hurt at all, just a bit surprised as she lay there in the grass with the scooter beside her. She looked up to the veranda where they were standing laughing. Eventually they came down and helped her. 'Hee-hee that was a bit of a flip!' was all they said.

She is thirteen when Frida Bertine is born. Her little sister likes to sit on her knee. 'Are you going to sit on Anne-Pia's knee when you are sixty too?' asks Peter.

Constance, who is no longer the youngest and who wants to show how grown up she is, looks seriously at Mum as she hangs up the phone after there is nobody on the other end. 'Perhaps it was someone who uses sign language?' she suggests.

The six children don't have specific chores to do around the house, but they have to keep their rooms tidy and, if they want to, they may cook a meal or bake. This means her too. She is often asked to babysit. Although she argues with her brothers and gets irritated by her sisters, who always want to come in her room, they are a comfort to her just by being there when she feels sad. It is with them she laughs the most. She doesn't think about it at the time but babysitting gives her responsibility and something other than herself to think about. Her siblings take her attention away from all the other things she thinks about.

Dead feet, what should I use them for? They dangle from the body, deathly pale, what do they want of me? What right do they have to demand that I take care of them? They are, and I am. We are two parts in one body. One part living and the other part dead.

When she is alone in her room her thoughts become short poems. That is how she can put words to her innermost feelings. Write herself away from the whirlwind of thoughts.

She now has some good thoughts about herself. Further education has opened up another world for her. Clubs, for instance. At Fakkelen club she is secretary on the board, she attends meetings and plans activities. Christian input and games. Pizza and pop. People. Friends. It is the social side that is the most important to her; the others can think about the Christian input. Of course she believes. She remembers Sunday school and the scare stories about hell. The thought of it causes her to believe. In this context it isn't so scary; hell pales into insignificance in relation to the new friends she has found. At least they can fear together.

In the last year of secondary school she is elected onto the school council. She gives a speech on the final evening. She shows what she is good for. Is strengthened.

He is one of those that can see right through her while other adults don't even see her. When you are fifteen a school taxi driver who's twenty is an adult. A lot of school taxi drivers have come and gone in her life. The faceless individuals pass her by, one by one. A regular occurrence every morning at just after eight, sometimes closer to half past eight, and again at two in the afternoon. They do their job and do it in silence, which suits her. It doesn't occur to her that it might be any other way. She can allow her thoughts to remain private, without a curious taxi driver trying to strike up a conversation.

She gets a new driver. He starts to chat to her. Not just the boring stuff like 'Hi/Bye' and the usual things that the others have managed to get out of her – he actually shows an interest in who she is. To begin with she thinks it will only last for the first couple of journeys. She feels like her thoughts have been invaded. He is curious about everything and he asks about things that have taken a long time to discuss even with friends. She suddenly has to consider herself in a new way; she cannot remain a good listener who doesn't put her feelings in the limelight. He is Socrates the philosopher who walked the streets of Athens and posed personal questions which helped those he met to understand themselves better.

This Socrates invades the safe space she has long occupied. That she has perhaps always occupied. Where everyone leaves her alone and do not demand that she be more than she dares to be when she has set her own limitations. She has only admitted to herself that she longs to be a normal teenager, and it is a deep sorrow that she cannot be. In that safe space nobody else knows that she carries that longing inside herself, so nobody pushes her. It is a safe existence but very lonely.

Along comes someone who wants to come in. Who tries to tempt her out without being aware of the part he plays in her life. He keeps talking, asking, commenting. He says she needs to be more forward with boys.

'They can be reserved about flirting with you, so you have to flirt and chat with them. Show them you are interested!'

'Naaa,' she replies and is relieved that they have parked outside her house and the conversation comes to an end.

Bit by bit she finds herself expecting him to chat to her, to be interested. To throw snowballs at her. They take a detour after school to drop off the other passengers first. She enjoys the attention because it is of a different sort to that which she usually gets from adults. This is about the girl inside her. He says the wheelchair does not affect the person you are.

In Year 9 at secondary school the end-of-year trip is, as usual, to Voss ski centre. A snow scooter and sledge have been arranged for her so she can enjoy the slopes like the others. She can have rosy cheeks, snow-wet clothes and cold fingers. She feels the joy of being the only one in control as she flies down the slopes. Steers the sledge with her arms, turns as she touches the slope, down, down, down as she leaves slightly worried teachers behind. For a few seconds she escapes from everything.

Dad and I have had an idea,' says Mum one day. They have come into her room to talk to her.

'You are a bit too heavy. You ought to try to follow a Greta Roede diet and cookery course. Everything would be much easier for you if you were a bit lighter.'

They are well-meaning parents who have no idea that I think about it all the time. That I struggle with myself because of the extra kilos which eat away at my self-confidence. Which means I disappoint them. Well-meaning parents who, when they said they wanted to talk to me, had no idea about my silent prayers as I fight the tears back: 'please don't let them say anything about my weight...'

'Dad and I have been thinking about something...'
Please, don't...
'...too many kilos...'
...don't...

She starts the diet. It goes surprisingly well with private follow-up from the course leader. Change the diet and more exercise. In six months she loses sixteen kilos. Summer arrives and her holiday to Beito. Everything slides. Good friends, food, drink. Food, food, food. She is back where she started.

I use a wheelchair. Wheelchair… user. I am dependant on a chair with wheels. It is my legs. I cannot stand on my own legs. I can't even feel them. I can't tell if they are cold. I am an invalid, handicapped, disabled, lame, a paraplegic. A wheelchair user… But first and foremost I am Anne-Pia.

I know what it is like to use legs. Once upon a time I could walk. I am now just a statistic. A stigmatized and categorized person. 'The disabled…' That's me. 'The disabled feel discriminated against…' That's me. 'The disabled have a lesser quality of life than others…' That's me. …But first and foremost I am Anne-Pia.

I sometimes feel down, yet other days I am fine.
It is horrible using a wheelchair.
The wheelchair doesn't matter to me.
Why should quality of life be dependent on whether one uses a wheelchair or not? The problem isn't the wheelchair but whether there are steps where you want to get to.
Using a wheelchair is not a problem
When it is Anne-Pia.

She really wants the good experiences to outweigh the horrible thoughts she has. She really is a happy girl. On the outside she manages to be the smiling and always-positive, brave girl, but gathering inside there is a lot of pain that won't let go and, at the same time, won't let her tell anyone. She has always managed to cope with these thoughts before, hasn't she?

She will manage now too.

She can't express her anger. Instead she becomes sad and upset. She lets the sad and upset come out when she is alone in her room.

The times when Mum and Dad see the sad upset girl they don't understand why. Nor can she explain it. There is never one specific situation that makes her feel that way, just a sudden hurt deep within her. Like an abscess that is leaking puss.

How does my failing body affect me? How am I affected when I feel that I have been pigeon-holed, not included because I can't walk?

She has always been a good girl. One who doesn't say anything or complain. In her situation she has developed an ability to care for others and their feelings and needs. She won't let her handicap get in the way of the needs and development of friends and families. She quietly accepts second place. She withdraws from situations that she cannot practicably take part in. She makes excuses for others and minimises problems. She is afraid that they won't like her any more and she is unconsciously afraid of not being friends with someone.

Now and then the inevitable happens and the repressed thoughts and feelings run over. They become unexplained crying and temper outbursts just because Mum and Dad won't let her do something she has planned to with Inghild. On these days she is thin-skinned and vulnerable. Everything that gets in her way - door frames, kitchen chairs, shoes, things she drops on the floor - fill her with hate, knock her off balance and to tears. Deep within herself she knows that she hates herself.

It is these thoughts that bubble up when she is out and about and something causes her to fall out of her chair. Her thoughts freeze but her brain is in overdrive when Dad comes towards her and the only thing she hears him say is her name in a critical way. 'Oh, Anne-Pia!' and her name sounds like a long critical pointing *what-have-you-done-now?* finger. In all the criticism she hears a frustrated *for-goodness-sake-think-about-what-you-are-doing* and an embarrassed *it-had-to-be-here-where-everyone-can-see.*

I hear all that in the way Dad says my name. I just want to escape from it all. Away from things I can't do. Away from people who stare. Away from Dad who pulls me up. Away from the criticism in my thoughts. I don't want to be here any more. I don't want to be me any more.

She has another battle within herself. To be able to have a relationship with her parents, both as a teenager, and as someone with a reduced mobility. A love-hate relationship. Other teenagers, who have no disability, feel that their parents don't understand, or aren't willing to put themselves in their teenager's place, and so don't let them have their own way. When that happens they can choose to distance themselves from their parents. Mum and Dad have to be part of her life. Every day. Several times a day. Mum and Dad help her to do things. They have to help her go to the toilet. It is them she has to rely on when she needs an errand running. The house feels like a prison, and the only escape is to withdraw further and further into herself, where all the thoughts she never shares with anyone lie in wait for her.

It is worst in the winter, when the snow is deep on the ground, because the car can't get up the steep hill. It has to park on the new road above the house. She needs the help of one or two people to drag her and her chair up the slope that runs from the back of the house up to the new road. She doesn't like it when people have to struggle to get her up to the car. Even though she doesn't have to do anything herself it is a struggle for her too. She feels so helpless and heavy. Nor does she like the feeling of sitting at home thinking that she can't go anywhere. It is binding not being able to go out whenever you choose, even though she may not have done it even if she could. The thought of not being able to, makes her feel it's unfair, hopeless, imprisoned. That makes her more sensitive. *You are so touchy. Don't take everything so personally*, she is told.

What happens inside me when I argue with someone I know I am totally dependent on? It is like the nightmare we have all had where we are running away from a monster and you realise you can't move. At best you move far too slowly – like wading through mud.

How can I get away from someone I can never escape from? What effect does it have on me when my common sense knows that it has to be this way at the same time as my heart and soul scream that it is wrong? Since I don't know why I think this way I can't show these thoughts for what they are. My helpers. My parents. The ones my body is getting ready to be separated from. The same body that is holding me back.

She doesn't make the connection between the feeling of grief and the fact that she feels sad and upset. Grief is when you've lost somebody you love, but she still has everyone. Grief can be a time when things aren't as good as they once were, but she's got all the help she could possibly need. Equipment, training, extension to the house – it's all meant to compensate for the life she should have had. It's all meant to make life good.

It doesn't occur to her that, when life changes so dramatically, you lose control over half your body, you can also feel grief. It's just like losing somebody you love. That nothing is the way it was before because dreams and hopes you had for the future have been lost.

She's never been able to put words to her sorrow. The sad Anne-Pia has never been taken seriously. She's always been cheerful, done her best, shown her happy, strong side so that people will be impressed. Nobody has known, important though it is, the price she's had to pay. It has cost her her soul. She's never said that she needs not to be strong and clever all the time. Her family and friends can't show her that they will love her just as much if she weren't always strong and clever.

Eventually, as time passes since the misdiagnosis, the reality of what has happened to her body disappears too. It was something that happened in the past. Life goes on. But she's spent a long time coming to the point where she acknowledges the effect it has had on the life she thought she would lead. The fact that it's in the past causes her to understate the extent of the consequences. Such as why she feels so different and hopeless and not able to cope in many situations. The fact that she ought to be glad because, despite everything, she has the full use of her arms. The fact that she ought not to feel ashamed because she's not able to do anything about her sad situation.

Therefore she finds it difficult to start a conversation every time she feels sad.

At sixth-form college she goes with the flow and chooses standard A levels. One morning, on her way to her place at the back of the classroom, Bente stops her.

'You know, *Mad, Mad World...*'

'Ye-ees ...'

Mad, Mad World is a magazine with articles from all over the world about the most unbelievable people. Everything from people who have become zombies or werewolves, to people who are haunted by monsters in the fridge. You suspect that a lot of the articles are made up, they seem too unbelievable to be true. She bought it once because she was curious about its content.

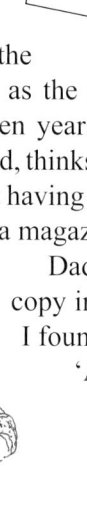

'Well,' continued Bente, 'you're in it!'

'What?!' For a moment she doesn't understand what Bente means.

'You're in the latest edition of *Mad, Mad World*!'

'No, no I'm not!'

'Yes, you are. But it says that you're seven...'

Bente gets a copy of it out of her bag and, sure enough, there is an article about her as a seven-year-old, with the cage. The article is exactly the same as the one in the Norwegian weekly magazine almost ten years ago. Stian, at the desk behind, thinks she should sue. She is surprised at having discovered herself in that sort of a magazine.

Dad comes home from work with a copy in his hand. 'Do you know what I found?'

'Already seen it,' she says.

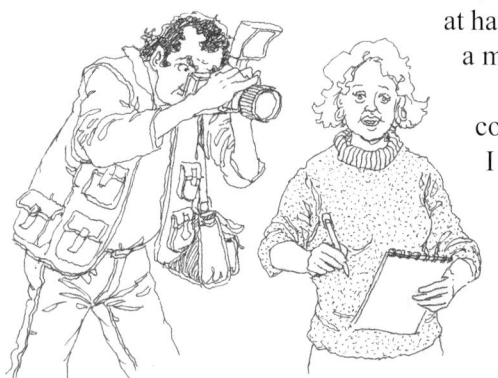

'NO TO THE EU' DEMONSTRATION

A trip is arranged to go to Oslo to take part in a demonstration against membership of the European Union (EU), in advance of the referendum about EU membership in 1994. In other words, you can get to the capital and home again, cheaply.

A group from her class are going on one of the buses. After several hours, the buses eventually arrive in Oslo. It's raining. A wet trip through the streets with the demonstration. The only thing she notices is how many stones and holes there are in the road, and she feels sorry for the people in the class who end up pushing her. She feels embarrassed and guilty when she needs a lot of help to be pushed in her wheelchair. A nuisance.

When the procession gathers in the square, politician Anne-Enger Lahnstein makes a speech against membership of the EU, but not much could be seen other than umbrellas. The only thing she can boast about is having heard Anne-Enger Lahnstein speak. One of the people beside her in the umbrella crowd, turns. In a motherly way, the lady comments about her lack of umbrella and sopping wet clothes. The lady says she'll get ill. She smiles back apologetically. After the official programme there's a couple of hours before the buses return home. Oslo City shopping centre is the next stop. She's not eaten since she left home. They don't get far inside the shopping centre before they notice a café, but they also notice the steps up to it.

'No problem,' declare her friends and, back-wheel first, they carry her step by step up. Half way up they notice that the other guests are staring at them. 'I don't suppose they've seen anyone in a wheelchair before and they're curious about what it is.' When at last she is safely up and her helpers are panting with relief, they turn and look at the other side of the café and suddenly realise why there were such a lot of people staring at them. If they'd gone round the side of the steps they'd just come up they would have noticed that the café has an excellent wheelchair ramp. Somewhat embarrassed and giggling they find a table. They have at least given the others some entertainment.

It's still a while until the bus heads back but she's already in her seat, ready for when the others come thundering in. She didn't come to protest. She's just glad that the bus driver hasn't complained at her because he had to carry her on board. She's had that happen to her before. So there she sits, reading comics alone in the bus whilst the others are still waiting outside. They wait as long as possible before taking their seats for the next seven hours. She can well understand it. She hears them chatting and laughing and suddenly recognises the feeling of being different again, although she's sure it wasn't their intention.

Imagine that I have to go to a psychiatrist because I have a breakdown in the classroom in the middle of a lesson. I suddenly begin to shout and scream and throw things. I almost expect that day to arrive, but nothing happens. I'm my usual self. Not all the days are as painful. The good days outweigh the bad and make me forget the painful ones. Until they come again.

When things get difficult she wants to run and hide from everything, somewhere where she can be cared for. This desire suddenly comes. Being admitted to hospital. Being so ill that she needs loads of attention. People attending to her, caring for her. And she can just receive, without doing anything, without thinking. To move into a thoughtless existence, three steps removed from reality, where pain, food and a dry and clean bed are the only things you need to relate to. It appears tempting, from a distance.

Poem by Anne-Pia, 16 years old

*Darkness comes
across my mind
covered with pain
wrapped around my soul.
Everything that's good
is gone.
If it has ever been?*

That's not the first time you've kissed,' he states, and leans back. It's not a question, and she's glad of the compliment. And she's not going to ruin it by saying that, actually, it is.

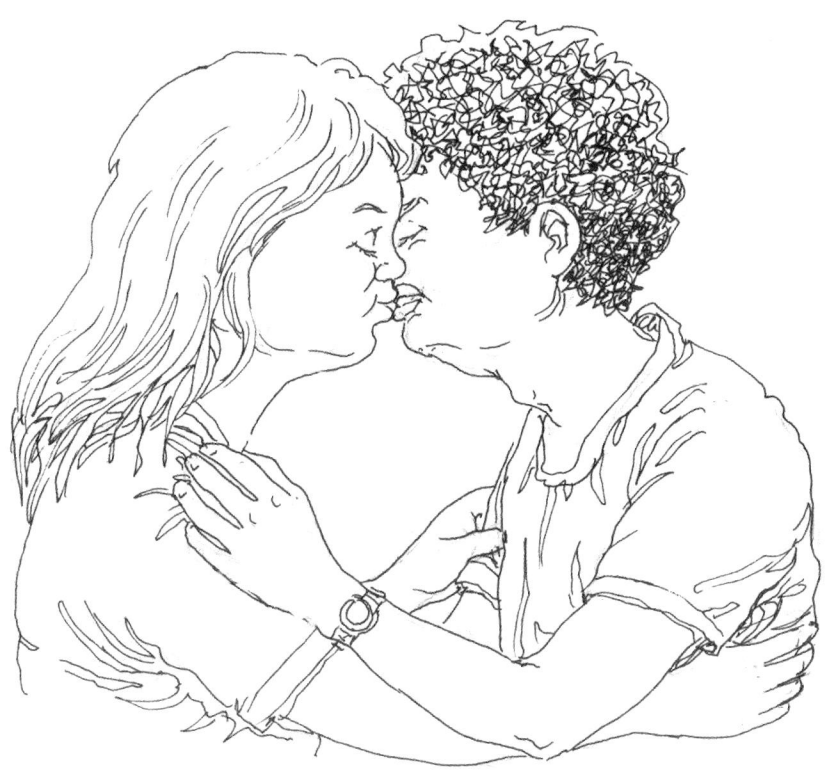

She and Inghild are part of a meditation circle. They explore alternative philosophies such as reincarnation, energy, intuition. They force her to ask questions that she's never asked before. Is God an old man who gets angry every time you say his name? Is it possible that he is within yourself? That he is the power that makes you more than you thought you could be, more than you think you are? Spiritually, they make strong new connections, but in all else they are pulling apart naturally, bit by bit, and although they are still good friends they are spending more and more time with other people. It's as though they have been for the other what they needed at the time and now they are ready to move on.

Nina comes into her life. They went to the same secondary school but didn't know about each other until Nina moved across to her class in the second year of A levels, and suddenly one day it's as though they have always been best friends. Did they first start to speak in the smokers' corner? Or in the classroom as mutual opposition to the teacher's worshipping of the cleverest pupils? When slowly but surely they couldn't be bothered and found other things to concentrate on?

Yet again she has found something in somebody who knows what it's like not to fit in. They both fit in to the small group who secretly smoke outside the library windows, where everyone who's going to or from the school has to walk past and can see that they are secretly smoking.

They can stand here and be looked at, with their cigarettes hidden in towards the wall or in their hand. But they look at the passers-by. Such as the actor Toralv Maurstad who is visiting his old stamping ground where he took his A levels. So much smaller and thinner are the white curls when you see them outside the TV screen.

If a teacher, employee or someone who knows your parents well or even maybe knows them, comes, you need to hide your cigarettes tight into the stone wall or behind your hand again. These breaks are the highlight of the school day. There are also free periods which are like breaks, and the odd school lesson where they sit a bit too long in a café and talk, smoke and eat the special Domus café pizza.

The academic aspects are not very important. She much prefers the time spent with her friends. She loves to feel like one of them, to be seen as the person she feels she is.

After having struggled with a urine infection and been ill a lot because of it, she gets a glimmer of hope up at Beitostølen as she talks to one of her friends up there. 'Why haven't you got a reservoir like me? It works really well. Makes life much simpler'.

This is new and interesting information. After talking to her doctor she applies for an operation to make an artificial bladder from part of her colon and redirect the ureters into it. It'll be much easier to empty it because you'll be able to do it through a hole in the stomach. There'll be fewer infections. The reservoir will also improve her quality of life because she'll be able to be more impulsive about trips and staying overnight. She'll no longer need a bench or bed. It'll just make everything so much simpler.

In the Autumn she is admitted to Førde Central Hospital. Not many people have had a reservoir operation like this. In Førde they've only ever done one before. It's arranged with the school that she'll be away for three weeks. It's her final year but they think she'll manage to catch up on her lost work. She's given a bed in a single room on the surgical ward. It has a TV. After the operation she's to remain there until she is secure with her reservoir and they see that it's working.

But things become more complicated than they anticipate and she ends up extending her stay. It's December and on 23 the entrance to the new bladder is suddenly blocked. She's taken down to theatre again for an emergency operation. She celebrates Christmas at the hospital but all celebration disappears in a cloud of queasiness and feeling unwell. Christmas dinner consists of re-heated porridge. She can't face being very sociable either and goes back to her room after the Christmas dinner. The family brings her some presents and the rest they save until New Year's Eve, when she comes home.

It's getting difficult to find any more places on her arm where she can be injected. The drip is put into a vein in her foot. So the vein can be used for as long as possible she has to sit still with her foot up on a stool. Three of her friends come with presents and good wishes from the class, but what really matters is that by doing so they show that they really do care. She thinks about everything that she's missed with her class, and she misses them all the more when they're there with her, and it makes her absence from the class more obvious. She should have been at her place in the classroom now, messing up Are's perfectly-styled hair and asking him to turn round so that they could do work together, alternately frustrated and amused in French with Nina, sitting at the back in English and listening to Hilde impressively reciting the American constitution off by heart in English.

We, the people of the United States, in order to form a more perfect union...

It's a huge contrast with the days that slowly pass here in the hospital. She can't face food. It just comes up again. In the end the only thing she can bring up is stomach acid.

The new operation doesn't lead to the new bladder functioning properly and they apply to transfer her to Haukeland Hospital in Bergen for a new operation. In the meantime she is to stay at home.

A STOMA THAT DOESN'T WORK

As a temporary solution she has a stoma bag fixed around the opening into her stomach so the urine can run straight into the bag. This doesn't work well for her. The whole thing gets wet, the urine runs around the edges where the bag is stuck to her skin and wets her clothes. In the middle of a lesson she might suddenly notice that the area is wet. She tries to hide it with her jumper which is already wet. When the lesson ends (she doesn't dare to draw attention to herself by going out in the middle of the lesson) she mumbles her apologies and hurries to the toilets to put layer upon layer of paper towels and toilet roll around the leak. If it is too obvious she has to ring the taxi company and ask them to come and collect her early. She innocently gives the driver the impression that they have been let out early, when she is on the edge of tears at the thought of someone having noticed her leak. The only thing to do is get home as quickly as possible and put on a new bag.

She joins in the celebrations in her final term of college as best she can. She was home just in time to see her year in their cabaret. She also joins in the mystery tour which includes bus, boat and two very early mornings waiting in the pouring rain for the bus. And there's a pyjama party, a party at the Fjaera pub and other parties in people's rooms. The stoma makes some things easier, but she is always afraid of leakage so that puts a damper on everything.

When she is with a boy at a party she doesn't think about what the stoma bag looks like on her body because it is, after all, only a temporary solution. The worst thing she can imagine is if the stoma bag comes unstuck or it starts to leak at the edges, and she ends up with urine everywhere. She convinces him not to go any further, when he obviously wants more. 'Can't we just carry on like this, sitting here and cuddling.' She appears calm on the outside, but she is petrified of leaks, her hand automatically checks the bag and she makes sure that he stays away from that area! She is glad when the bag keeps all the liquid in until she gets home.

She is spending all her energy at the moment in worrying about the stoma bag, but not only that. As well as the stoma there is, as there has always been, all the practical matters that she needs to plan in her head such as toilet, steps, house…

But those times when she allows herself to lose control, not to have an overview of everything, she generally finds that things work out fine. As a rule the problems are worse in her mind than in reality. It is in these moments that she feels like a normal teenager. The final year of school has been one of the best and worst rolled into one.

At Haukeland hospital she has the operation she was originally supposed to have had. Without complications. But her kidneys have been affected.

Afterwards, the stoma bags and equipment can be thrown away. She can now empty herself more easily than ever, using disposable catheters attached to a bag. She has a skin-coloured plaster covering the opening in her stomach. As long as she empties her bladder every three hours, or more or less often depending on how much she drinks, she has no leakage problems.

She has got her much-desired car, two years after sending in the application for it. She can now focus on taking her driving test. Thanks to the car she becomes even more independent. The car is much used in her second final year. She has to repeat her final year of college since she had missed so much.

Another major thing that helps her that year, is her role in the group for six-year-olds which has just begun. Frida Bertine is in it. The children are very pleased every time she drives into the college and gets herself out using the automatic lift at the back of the car. The fact that she is about to leave college, with all the ritual that involves in Norway, makes her seem all the more exciting. They make waffles indoors, read books, play, and Ingrid the teacher shows them how to make Indian webs using ice-lolly sticks and thread.

Far Away

When much of your life is spent in the health service, it is like sitting on the side-lines of your own life. You cannot always decide what is best for yourself. It has been a big step to suddenly find herself over eighteen, and that the automatic support of the health service is not the same as it was when she was legally a child.

Once she has finished sixth form she wants to get far away. To somewhere nobody knows her. Far enough away to show everyone that she can manage alone. None of the further education colleges she rings are able to accommodate wheelchair users. She doesn't want more daily challenges about this. Her primary school had to be converted for her, as did her secondary school, and the further education college. This time she wants to choose a college which is perfect from the start. She takes the negative replies as a sign, a sign to choose unconventionally.

Janne and she start at West Jutland College, in Denmark.

It is snowing and they have just got off the airport bus at Oslo Central Station. They wait outside, surrounded by suitcases and boxes full of presents, and wonder how to find the bus they need for the rest of their journey.

'We first need to find something to put our baggage on so we can take it with us!' Janne heads towards the huge staircase, 'I'll be back in a moment with a trolley!'

She sits there in the snow, in the midst of all the boxes and suitcases. She tries to look worldly wise and not lonely.

Don't look people in the eye. Look after the baggage. Don't think that all those around you are potential murderers who see at a glance that you are helpless and alone. Where has Janne got to? There is a man standing smoking over there; he's looking this way! Don't look at him. Act like you are waiting for a big muscle-man who is just around the corner. What do you do when waiting for someone who is only 'round the corner'?

Oh no, he really is looking over here, he's coming this way! Oh no, horrible old man, go away! I have no money, just Christmas presents! How could you dare to steal from someone surrounded by baggage in a wheelchair in the snow?

Go away!

He really is coming here. Look down, don't make eye contact. Look down at the white snow. Don't think about the knife that will soon glisten in his right hand which has just thrown away the cigarette and which even now is reaching deep into his coat pocket.

'How can I identify him for the police if I don't look at him?' she wonders. The only thing she has noticed is that he has white hair. Perhaps I should glance up and have a good look at him so I get the details right? He is now beside her.

'You shouldn't stand out here with all that baggage.'

'I am waiting for someone, she'll be back in a moment, she has just gone to find a luggage trolley.'

'It is not safe. I can wait with you. I am waiting for someone too.'

So they wait together, the possible murderer and her. Janne appears, rushing with the trolley, and the murderer helps load the trolley and get it into the station. Before he disappears to find the person he is expecting, he tells them where to go.

'Have a good journey, good luck!'

'Thanks for your help!'

'What a nice man!' says Janne.

'Yes,' she replies.

DEPRESSION?

Velling, Denmark, 17 January 1998

Everything feels dark and empty. Everyone has got it in for me. I say almost nothing. Have withdrawn into myself. I think about suicide but don't want to live this life again. Everyone is content with themselves and with others. I feel stupid. Nobody cares about me or even notices me. I don't want to say anything. Nobody hears me anyway and when I say nothing I am stupid. I hate it when people say 'you're quiet today...?'

I have no energy. Why am I like this? I want to get out of here, to feel pleasure and joy and love. I'll leave after the trip to Hungary. Can't leave before because G has worked so hard to make it possible for me to go.

I don't want to go home. Yes, but only for a little while. I want to go places. Am restless. Want to sleep. Away from myself and my thoughts.

She is pleased when things work out in a way that means she can go on the college trip to Hungary. When they get to the hotel, she cannot get into the bathroom. They are meant to be staying there for several days! After twenty-one hours on the bus with very little sleep, her feelings overwhelm her. Janne sits beside her and tries to comfort her. When some of the adult ladies on the trip get to hear about the situation, they come into her room to talk to her. They offer to help her every morning and evening. In this way she sees Hungary as more than just a problem.

A couple of days after they get back to college Henry wants to talk to her. 'We think you should throw a party as a thank-you to the people who helped you in and out of the bus.'

'Who is the "we" that all think that?'

'They don't think you are very thankful.'

'Are they upset with me?'

'Yes, they think you are ungrateful.'

'But I have thanked them! I thanked them every time they helped me in and every time they carried me out. What more can I say? If I had to arrange a party every time someone helps me I would never do anything else!'

'I just thought I would mention it, as a friend.'

They buy in the ingredients. Janne has a recipe for a spice cake. The plan is to say at dinner time that all those who were on the Hungary trip, and helped her, are to gather in a room after dinner.

But time is short, their program is full. They don't ever get that far. It is weighing on her conscience. It has quietened a bit since Janne said she should pay no attention to what Henry said. Inside herself, she wonders whether there is some truth in Henry's words, whether she really is egoistic and ungrateful. That she does not manage to show how much she appreciates all the help she gets. Is it the shame of feeling that she is always a burden that gets in the way? Is there some unspoken rule of which she is unaware?

Henry's mother is a teacher in a junior school. She is asked whether she would help some of the pupils. Year 4 are having a project and two of the girls have been asked to investigate what it is like to be disabled. Of course she will help and soon afterwards she receives a hand-written letter from the girls with questions for her to answer. They will use it as the basis for their project. There are questions about how it happened, whether she has a job, whether she can do things others cannot do. She answers as honestly as possible. She likes being asked.

A few days after sending in her reply she receives a thank-you note with a picture and drawings.

During the Easter holidays, she, Janne, and Claus travel around Denmark in her car. He wants to show them the little house in Lolland where his friend, the dog and the rabbits in the outdoor cage are, as well as the flat in Copenhagen.

It is strange and good at the same time. Sleeping on a mattress on the floor, high up in a flat in Copenhagen. Being woken by a Dane creeping in to wake her. Lies beside her, close. Lying there cuddling until it is time to get up. In the sitting room, feeling him around her. His breath. His smell. At times like this, it feels like the stories she reads in magazines. Yet this is better because it is happening to her and nobody can take it away from her.

At times like this she doesn't associate her body with illness – quite the reverse. Now it is desirable. It has a new identity.

When she was a child she had to relate to her body in a different way to healthy children. Everyone who touched her body did so because they had to check something, wash it, inject it, cut it, bandage it, stick needles in it to see if she could feel anything.

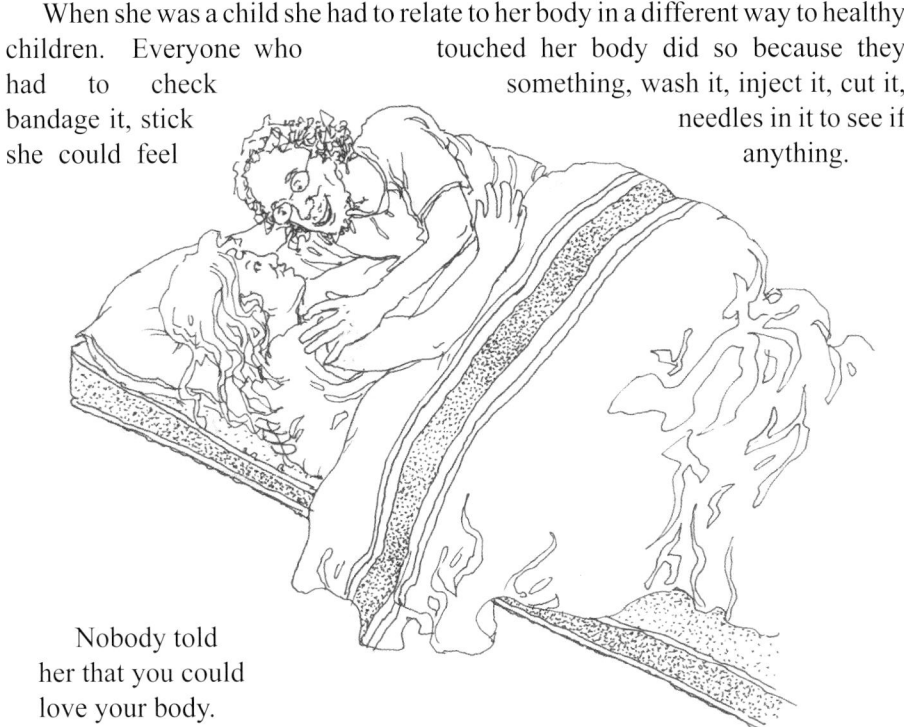

Nobody told her that you could love your body.

Monday 1 July 1998

I HATE it when Dad drops hints about my weight. I have been home for a month and everything has been fine. I didn't think it would be too bad at home this time – until he said it would be a good idea to go on a diet before going to college.

I went to the bathroom and tried to make myself sick. It feels like someone has pulled a plug out of me. All the self-confidence I have worked on building up, and the time spent learning to love myself during those seven months in Denmark, has just disappeared. Everything is the same as it always has been. I am ugly, fat and stupid again. I am angry because I am always asked to baby-sit and angry with myself for being angry about it. I love my sisters – it is just the principle of it! Also that 'everyone' uses my car; although it is selfish to say no because I don't use it very often, I really shouldn't always be lending it out…

I am going to have to start smoking again!!!

SOGNDAL

She spends a year studying English at Sogndal College. Just like the previous year she rings all the colleges in the country to ask if they are able to accommodate wheelchairs. She ought really to visit each college to be certain, but instead she has to rely on them telling the truth and make her decision based on that.

The next thing is to contact the bursar and enquire as to whether they have accommodation for wheelchair users and hope she is allocated a place in one of them as there is a shortage of such rooms.

It is like detective work in a jungle and she would love to have help from someone who could advise her. Someone with a list of the right contacts. Someone who could take over when the jungle had used up all her energy. When she was part of a system that decided and made plans it made some things much simpler. But living life within the health service also means living life from the sidelines. She did not decide what was best for her. If she was asked but didn't really know what she thought, the others could say what they thought was best.

To be eighteen and therefore an adult is not always so simple, because the health service has now fulfilled its responsibility towards her. She is suddenly solely responsible for her health and her future. It is up to her now. She meets official opinions and assumptions without any experience in dealing with them alone. Facing the world without anyone to watch her back.

I look down at my body. A mistake took my legs away from me and I will never walk, feel the sand between my toes, jump or dance. A mistake that was out of my control. But I am the one who is letting my body and soul deteriorate, who locks all the painful thoughts deep within myself and feeds them with false comfort. I allow it to happen. I cannot see that it is happening. I turn away from myself and look the other way. I do this because I am convinced that I know best how to help myself, without involving others. This is what is called repression. Repressing the fact that I am not OK. Repressing the fact that I need help. Repressing myself whilst at the same time thinking about nothing but myself – just in the wrong way. In a way that doesn't help. Without love towards myself. If I had love for myself I would not have allowed these thoughts and actions.

The bed-sit is at the top of a hill. If it snows in the winter and gets slippery it will be impossible to get down in the car. She has a converted Volkswagen

153

Caravelle with a hand-operated accelerator and a brake at the side of the steering wheel. Nina is studying to be a nursery nurse in the same village. The bed-sits are some distance apart but they visit each other as often as they can.

She quickly gets to know the others in her class and goes out with them now and then. It feels so empty when she doesn't have any visitors or isn't out visiting others. She closes herself away in her bed-sit more and more. She buys crisps as comfort food when she is alone. When she is out she makes excuses to come home and eat. Whenever she has eaten she feels guilty, feels really bad, and so she tries to make herself sick. When someone comes to visit, she sits there wondering when they will go so she can grab more crisps which she, almost secretly, bought at the shop. Every time she buys sweets or other treats to eat, she does it with a guilty conscience and wonders what the shop assistants must think of her.

During the semester there will be a three-week trip to York. She spends a lot of time discussing with her teachers to what degree the college they will be visiting is wheelchair accessible. They decide that she is to stay a short distance away from the others in another building. It's not known whether she will be able to get into the bathroom and shower. Despite this, she wants to go on the trip. One regrets things one has not done, more than those things one has done.

On the morning of the flight from Sogndal I panic. What if I can't shower or wash myself for three weeks? What if I am not included in the social activities because I am staying in a different building? Will I cope and not totally exhaust myself? I weigh up the one thing against the other, make up my mind then change my mind again and again. I have not been to England and it will be an experience. I have coped with this sort of problem before.

'I'm going!'
'No, I daren't take the chance.'
'I'm going!'

Her class are waiting for her at the airport when her teacher rings.
'Where are you?'
'I am sorry, I am not coming. I daren't risk it.'

The following year she starts and finishes studying for a teaching qualification at Volda University College. It takes all the energy that ought to be spent on her studies to plan and organise so that she will be able to function on a practical daily level. The constant feeling of not quite 'getting there' eats away at her self-confidence. With no energy and a low self-image she doesn't join in the social side of student life. She asks the local authority for a support person for the current academic year, but it creates a situation that she is not at ease with. Someone who is paid to be her friend. She attends a number of student activities alone, chats to people but feels alone.

It ends in her breaking off her studies and moving back home to her parents, where she has a work placement as a classroom assistant in the local school. She doesn't know what she wants to do with her life. She develops stress-related pain in her shoulders. During a visit to the doctor she is asked what she is filling her time with at the moment.

'What career do you want to follow?'

'I think I might like to work with pupils who need extra help and support.'

'No, that will be difficult. You mustn't imagine that children with special needs will want to have a teacher who uses a wheelchair. It is hard enough for them as it is.'

'Noooo.'

Mum is waiting outside when she returns to the car. She looks down but can't manage to hide her red eyes and the tears that just keep falling. She needs to get away from there before she can begin to explain about the doctor's appointment. After that she knows even less what she wants to do with her life.

She is determined to get an education regardless of what she is told she can't do for a career. She reads through the information in the college prospectuses about subjects in which she is interested, applies and is offered a place to study Scandinavian languages at Kristiansand College.

She has again applied to a college which is far from home. She tries to begin again in a place where nobody knows her. A clean start. She moves into student accommodation. On her first day she gets into conversation with someone else who lives there. She thinks that it will be fine this time. In the class there are people of all ages, which is exciting. It doesn't take long for her to meet Marianne, who has just moved here with her husband and three-year-old daughter. They 'adopt' each other as sisters.

She applies to work in the student radio station and joins in various organised activities. She tries to build up a broad social network. She finds herself a physiotherapist and a cleaner for her bed-sit. The thing about moving to a new place is that she doesn't know what support the local authority offers or whom to get in touch with.

She sorts everything out, puts things in place so she can enjoy being a student. She does however feel unwell when she goes out shopping or for a walk in her electric wheelchair. It seems like everyone stares at her disparagingly. She knows she would cope better with it if there was someone with her but she doesn't know anyone in the area. Marianne lives out of town and she only meets the others during class or at the radio studio.

After one programme, the group from the radio are going into town for a party. She can feel a knot inside her. She would really love to go with them but explains that she needs to be up early in the morning because she is expecting to take delivery of a bed. The others say that is no problem as they too have to be up early. She panics and insists that she needs to go straight home. She is not being honest with them; the bed is coming later in the day but she doesn't know them well enough to tell the truth, that she is afraid of being left out. There will almost certainly be steps up to where they are going and since she has come to work in her electric chair, which is too heavy to be lifted up steps, she would need to go home and swap chairs. She is sure they would not wait until she had done that. If she is to be coming home late at night she would need to take her car since it can be difficult to find a taxi so late. If she is driving she can't drink and *that* wouldn't be right either since they are going partying. If she drinks she needs to go to the toilet and she knows from experience that she can't always get in to public toilets. It is OK if she has one drink – that doesn't make her need to wee. Then there is the taxi home. She would need to get into a telephone box and she doesn't know the number of any taxi companies. It might be that they go somewhere that she cannot get to and she loses them and is left alone in an unknown city. In the middle of the night. She has to get up for the bed delivery.

It is too much to explain all that on the first time they are going out together so she insists again that she really does have to be up for the bed. They give up in the end and she heads home while the others head for the night life. The following day they tell her about stopping a bus to take them into town. '*That's how far I would have managed to keep up with them,*' she thinks, relieved that she decided to go home.

The college is on an old military camp, so the classrooms are spread around the campus in various cabins. She uses her electric chair and is able to move about without assistance. Only one of the cabins has a big enough toilet and that means a lot of to-ing and fro-ing, especially when she is dealing with the effects of many cups of coffee with Marianne. Marianne has her flask of coffee with her everywhere, and opens it both in the breaks and in the lessons.

She uses her car to get to college. When winter arrives with its ice and snow she sits in the car with the engine on and the heater blowing to defrost the windscreen as she cannot scrape the ice off by hand. She has not grasped how the heater works. If someone appears from the building she sometimes asks them to scrape the windscreen for her so she doesn't arrive late every day. Getting up any earlier is not an option. It is not an ideal solution but it worked in Sogndal so it can work here too.

She finds a note with information about the student chaplain. She has never been to see a member of the clergy, or anyone else. She keeps the note safe and, a couple of days later, gets in touch. She talks about how she feels that everything is stressful because so much energy is spent on practical matters and on worry which leaves her unmotivated for her academic work. She can't hold the tears back as she talks. She has a couple more sessions with the student chaplain.

I am noticing more and more that things aren't as I had imagined they would be. Instead of being part of the student life where I live, I close myself off in my room. I unconsciously make excuses for not going up to the communal TV room. Instead I watch TV alone. I often eat. I imagine what it would be like if I went up there, that the others have already met and formed groups. That I won't have anyone to talk to and will feel stupid. No, it is safer to stay here.

On one occasion she dares to go up. There is a note on the entrance door which says there's to be a party and everyone is invited. That evening she puts on her make up and party clothes. She has butterflies; it is now or never. Two minutes after she arrives she realises that this is not for her. There are very few people there, and at the table where she sits they say almost nothing. People only chat to those they came with. It seems that everyone except her has come with others. She stays as long as she feels she must, then mumbles something about having realised she has forgotten something or needs to go to the toilet, leaves the table and goes out of the door.

Into the freedom of the hall. It was certainly only the people who had to get up to let her past who noticed that she left. She rolls back down to her room. To the TV. To food.

When she meets people in her accommodation block, in the laundry room or in the hallways, they are pleasant towards her but nevertheless it doesn't encourage her to go up the TV room again. When she goes home for her summer break she promises herself that, when she returns for the autumn term, she will dare. When she thinks about it while at home it doesn't seem like such a difficult thing to do.

When she returns to continue her studies the new college building is completed and in use, with everyone based in the same building. Everything will be much easier now. She soon discovers that for those who are dependent on the lift there is always a detour to get back and forth, up and down.

If you can walk up the stairs it is easy to arrive exactly where you need to be, but she has to go along a long corridor to the lift. Out of the lift and along another long corridor to the classroom. This means that breaks go very quickly. It curbs her social activities as she cannot pop to the canteen with the rest of her class. Fortunately Marianne is willing to take the detour with her.

She wakes in the morning feeling ill. It is as though all her energies have been sucked out during the night. All the negative thoughts that she struggles with in the evenings and at night are inside her, making her feel sick and her eyes to overflow. She takes the day off sick. Gets up late, does some homework with breaks to watch TV. Eventually, as the day trundles on, she wonders if it was a mistake not to go to classes. Might she manage to go out anyway? She would probably feel better in a while. Just think, the others will be sitting in the canteen now, chatting and enjoying themselves. They are a nice group. She feels good when she is with them. She could be sitting there now laughing with them. Is it too late?

She glances at the clock and feels guilt overwhelm her. She has missed so much today. Her thoughts bring her back to reality. The reality of the four white walls and the door separating her from the others. Out there, where she cannot face being. Perhaps tomorrow.

She and Marianne go on a trip to revise for their exams. They head first to

Denmark and rent a cabin by the sea; next year to a campsite in Sogn. They cover the walls with sheets of paper full of grammatically-correct sentences, metaphors, weak and strong verbs, pronouns, adjectives, masculine, feminine and neuter words, authors, relevant dates and language reforms.

They must learn everywhere; the toilet, the kitchen, in their sleep almost. When they are not studying they discuss their studies. They discuss while making dinner, over a glass of red wine, in their breaks. They compare all that they see and all that they talk about. Swedish, Danish, Norse, Henrik Wergeland and Amalie Skram's poems, Ivar Aasen's travels collecting local dialects.

Being at home with Marianne and her little family saves what remains of her. The laughter is like a fountain of water that fills her and nourishes her through the difficult jungle. It strengthens her.

So why did she go home after the second year? She has passed all her exams, she has friends but she is restless. She is alone too much. It is difficult to deal with her self-image which is becoming smaller and smaller. She gives up in the end and while talking to her Mum she says she is moving back home.

Nothing comes of her brave plan to spend more time in the TV room. The evening before she leaves there for good, she dares to go in but only because her TV is packed into her car. She gets into a conversation with two lads about the new *Lord of the Rings* film.

'I haven't seen you up here before?' says one of them in surprise.

'No,' she replies, but cannot come up with a good reason as to why not and so tries to change the subject.

If only she had landed in this situation the last time she dared to come up here. Could everything have been different?

They are pleased to have her home. She discovers that Dad wants her to be more active in political life. It is difficult to get young new people. She can feel her opposition throughout her body but at the same times feels she has no choice.

'You are disabled and so it should be you fighting for things.'

She is elected onto the county board for the disability association for two years.

It is as if a final judgement has fallen for her. She cannot escape it. By doing this she has put herself in a position that no normal person wants. That is the way she feels about it.

She doesn't get the chance to be normal. This makes her angry but she can't express her thoughts. Nobody would understand why she would not want to be involved in something that is about her and her group. That would just make her into an unthankful egoist. She will benefit from this. It is for her own good.

It is the other people on the board that turn this into a good experience for her. It is the people they are, the way they act, the tasks for which she is given responsibility, the members of the team, the life experiences she is able to share that turn her negative preconceptions into positive experiences. She still doesn't like politics but in retrospect sees the positive things that she's taken part in, been a part of.

It is no better in her private life. She buys a flat in town which needs renovating and converting. It is so she can have her own space, which she can rent out if she decides to move back home. She has to live at home until the work is completed.

She feels squeezed in all directions, expectations which come both from within and from outside her.

'What are your plans?'

'Are you going to get a job?'

'Are you back for good?'

Failure. Fat. Coward. Might as well just disappear. I will never amount to much.'

Her summer job at the travel agent's and her job at directory enquiries seem, from the outside, to be going fine, but she is ill at the thought of everything that she mustn't do wrong. She thinks over situations again and again to find out what she said and did, and what she could have said or done better. She has nightmares because she thinks that, if she can't tackle this, she'll just be proving what many people already believe; that people with a handicap are of a lower order than others. The doctor at Sunnaas, who himself used a wheelchair, had told her that they had more to prove, so it was even more important to get a good education. To be above average.

Just at the moment it feels as though she is comprehensively pulling down the average.

I run my fingers over my upper body to try and find out where the boundary goes between where I have feeling in my skin and where I don't. The boundary is unclear. Some places I can't feel anything. I panic at the thought that the paralysis might be spreading up my body and that in the end I will be completely paralysed.

But the neurologist says it is difficult to know if that could happen since I don't know whether I have had feeling in any of those places before.

'It probably won't happen now after so many years,' he says.

DISQUIET

Thursday afternoon

She feels disquiet in her body. It starts with the phone ringing. She doesn't answer it in case it is work ringing. Her job at directory enquiries means that she is sometimes rung at short notice and asked to work. For no reason in particular she has no desire whatsoever to go into work today. She assumes it is one of her periods of depression starting. She doesn't bother looking who is ringing. She doesn't bother answering the phone.

Friday morning

She is woken by the phone ringing again. She reaches out and grabs the mobile from beside her bed. When she notices that the number is work, she ignores the ringing.

Why?

She has the same feeling of disquiet today as well but much stronger. The phone stops ringing. Starts ringing again. And stops. It rings a third time… and a fourth… She puts the phone on silent and drops it into the bag on the back of her wheelchair.

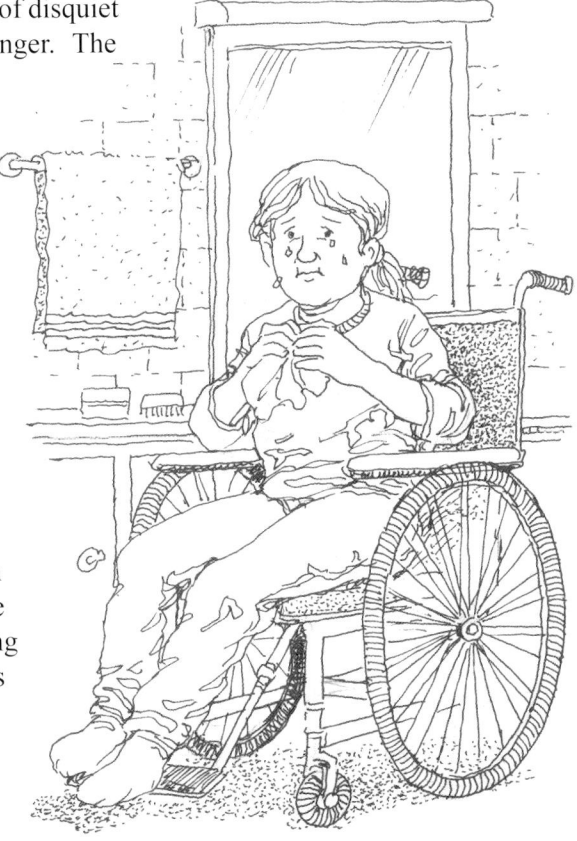

She gets dressed and up into her chair. Rolls to the bathroom. Doesn't feel like talking to anyone today. The disquiet weighs heavily on her. Suddenly she is in the bathroom with tears rolling down her face. She sits there in the bathroom and cries for an hour.

What *is* going on?

A little while later the doorbell rings. She wipes away her tears. It's Mum. 'I bought some tea lights for you as we used yours up at the party,' says Mum as she comes in. She takes the parcel and puts it in the drawer while she does everything she can to appear normal. She fails and the tears start again.

'What is the matter?' Mum looks at her in concern.

'I don't know,' she says, truthfully. 'I just started crying... I don't feel right... I am not OK...' The words stumble out between her sobs.

I don't know what is going on. I have always been so good at hiding it when I am sad. I have at least never admitted that I am sad, or sobbed in front of Mum in this way. The family have never gone in for talking about how we are. I have never been able to talk to anyone about it when I am not feeling good. I have found it embarrassing. I want my Mum and Dad and brothers and sisters to think that I can tackle anything.

'It must be the final straw which breaks the camel's back,' she thinks, and actually feels a bit relieved. Now that, at last, Mum has seen her like this she asks her Mum to do something that she knows she won't do herself. She asks her to ring the doctor. She wants to be referred to a psychiatrist.

The same day she packs a few things and goes home with Mum. She can't face being alone. The rest of the day is in a cloud. She doesn't manage to either smile or laugh. She is just sad. She isn't really part of anything. Luckily her brothers and sisters are out a lot of that day so she can be peaceful in her own world.

Night falls. At about two in the morning she goes to bed. She gets out her mobile which has been turned off since the morning. Several texts land. The first is from Nina who is on a work placement in Oslo and wants to know Inghild's surname. She replies to the message before opening the next one. From Peter. 'Have you heard about Inghild?' She doesn't understand and opens the next message. It is from Ragnhild. 'Isn't it terrible that they can't find Inghild?' Something about the choice of words in both messages makes her realise that this is serious. A thought makes her go back into the sitting room and turn on the teletext. One of the headlines grabs her:

Norwegian Inghild (25) feared dead in Africa

Her hands are shaking as she turns to the page with more of the story. A boat has capsized in Africa on Thursday night. There was a Norwegian woman on board. Inghild. Many dead. Many missing. Feared dead.

The last time she saw Inghild was six months ago, with Nina, at an alternative therapy fair in Bergen. Inghild was on a stand giving massages. Inghild with her warm hands. They had been thrilled to see each other again. It had been a long time. Inghild had invited them to a party that evening. They didn't go.

She hears someone in the bathroom. Through her tears she shouts for Mum because she assumes it is her. It is Guro. Her sister comes in. She points at the TV, unable to say anything. Guro reads the screen. She automatically grabs Guro's hand and hangs on to it. 'Should I get Mum?' asks Guro. Without waiting for an answer she rushes off to get her. Mum comes at once. They stay there and talk. Tears fall. 'She might be alive? She must be!' A day later her body is found. Her soul has gone home.

Almost two weeks after her death, Inghild's family can hold her funeral. She is asked to sing *The Rose* in church. She can remember Inghild singing it often. She liked it very much. She remembers all the times they have sung together. Of course she will. It will be her way of saying farewell. In the church and at the hotel where they hold the wake, Inghild's paintings are on display. The previous year Inghild had secretly recorded a CD of songs which she had given to her family for Christmas. They play some of the songs at the funeral. At the wake Inghild's mother reads some of Inghild's emails. The emails describe the project with which she is involved in Africa. That her gift with her warm hands got stronger and stronger. That the African way of life has much to teach us. How strong the energy is there and she hopes the pain is behind her now.

The boat that Inghild was travelling on sank Thursday night 26 to 27 September. The day she died was the day of my breakdown. All the thoughts and feelings inside me pushed their way to the surface and led to me being able to talk to someone.

And this time I didn't say that everything was fine.

'A Warrior of the Light needs love.

'Love and affection are as much a part of his nature as eating and drinking and
a taste for the Good Fight. When the Warrior watches a sunset and feels no joy, then
something is wrong.

'At this point, he stops fighting and goes in search of company, so that they can
watch the setting sun together.

'If he has difficulty in finding company, he asks himself: 'Was I too afraid to approach someone? Did I receive affection and not even notice?

'A Warrior of the Light makes use of solitude, but is not used by it.'

From *Warrier of the Light*, a manual, by Paulo Coelho

All is not made well by waving a magic wand. Many small steps are needed when there is a lot to come out into the open, be looked at and repaired.

It is exhausting work, finding yourself. Believing in yourself. Having new thoughts about yourself.

Her body brings up all the painful experiences and thoughts. Everything is to go!

Away!

Sickness in body

The following year is spent fighting through the deep darkness of my own mind.

When eventually I make it to the surface, my body turns against me, allowing pockets of infection to develop inside me. I arrive at Førde Hospital with a temperature of 40.5 degrees Celsius. I am shivering so much that the bed shakes, despite two duvets, several blankets and hot water bottles around me. 'We need to put a permanent catheter in your stoma!' explains the nurse, and I start to cry in panic reliving the previous time when there was something wrong with the stoma here in this same hospital.

The nurses stayed with me through the reaction, comforted me, and calmed me down, and to my huge relief they managed to insert the catheter without any problem. A week went by and they wanted to send me to Haukeland Hospital in Bergen.

It was at the worst possible timing. Mum had been with me all morning and had gone into town for shopping. They came into my room and said that the air ambulance was ready to take me. Sorry, there is no time to lose, they might be called to another job at any time and then it will be too late. No, Mum doesn't have a mobile. She will be back soon.

We left before she came.

Mum came back to the ward to find an empty bed and a wheelchair left behind. She ran into the corridor shouting. Someone came and explained what had happened. It was the worst possible timing. I lay in the helicopter, supported by pillows so I could see out, down on the mountains, while I thought about how poor Mum will react when she returned to the ward. I arrived in Bergen thirty-five minutes later. I had an intravenous drip and my body was filled with strong antibiotics. A *no-messing* huge dose they called it.

My infection count was over four hundred. It should normally be about ten. It was too risky to operate because of my anatomy. My organs are much too close to each other. Squashed together in my short upper body. The infection count had to be reduced with medication and by what they could drain out using needles and catheters into the pockets of infection. It was in my liver, kidneys and blood and the procedure had only been tried a few times b e f o r e . The doctors were afraid of accidentally damaging my good kidney or lungs. After one draining procedure I had problems breathing and had to be given oxygen. I couldn't draw my breath in deeply because of pain and breathing difficulties. I only just had enough breath to speak in sentences or to hold a phone conversation. On one occasion I had to hang up.

Lots of people rang. Lots sent flowers. Some came to visit. They showed that they cared. I was in Haukeland Hospital for two months, and at one point I didn't even have the energy to sit up in bed. I thought I would never manage to get back to the fitness level I had previously. I did, though! It took four months with home help. With training. With Constance and Frida Bertine taking turns to sleep over with me so they could help me into my chair in the morning. Four months before I once again managed alone.

That autumn I moved to Bergen to complete my education but, if Ragnhild had not been with me when I moved, taken control, organised and encouraged, I would have given up. It was another difficult period of provision which didn't work and help that didn't materialise. I couldn't manage without help in the student room I was allocated. It was thirty degrees outside and the catches to open the windows were out of my reach at the top. The fridge door opened the wrong way so I could not fit between it and the wall when I wanted to use the fridge. After some discussion I was allowed to move to a more suitable room where I could manage alone. When we asked for help to move my bed down four floors the caretaker said he did not have time to do it. 'We have to carry in sandwiches for the press conference about the new student flats and we are expecting the mass arrival of several thousand students.'

'What do you suppose I am?'

If I had been alone in that situation I dare not think about how I would have been. Ragnhild was there and she was angry on my behalf about that and similar situations. She said she could not believe what she had just heard. I knew then that it wasn't me there was something wrong with. That made the world of difference. Where a system had again labelled my identity as 'sickness' and, on top of that, made me feel worthless, this caused her as an individual to respond in the opposite way. She supported my healthy identity by meeting bureaucratic attitudes alongside me and because she reacted to them.

GOOD EXPERIENCES

It was more important than ever to fill the autumn with good experiences. Nina and I went to the alternative therapy fair in Oslo. The four eldest of us siblings, who were now spread around the country, went together to a concert, also in the capital, and heard the German band Rammstein. Only a few short months ago I would not have thought I could do any of these things. At that time I needed help to get in and out of bed, and help from the district nurse to have a shower and get dressed.

After I started to be thankful for everything, being glad even for the smallest things I can find to be thankful about, I have changed my attitude. I find new things to be thankful for every day. I am so fortunate to be able to live in Bergen and still have my home in Sandane. That I have a good relationship with my brothers and sisters. That I am allowed to study. That I can get to know good people. When things don't go well I have had help from unexpected places. I have my car and the Balder electric wheelchair that I finally was able to get...

All of this means that I appreciate every day and has a positive effect on the way I interact with others. It is a privilege!

THE JOB CENTRE

I had already accepted the university place, so the plan was that, after Christmas, I would study in a different faculty. But a week before my preliminary exams, a week before the Christmas holidays, I received a phone call from social services and was told I could not study any more - or at least not with any form of economic support from them.

I should of course have remembered that they will only give support for three years. Of course I could carry on studying – take out a student loan and grant as others have to do. But my body and my soul objected. Could not take any more. After the exams I packed my things and moved back home. Sometimes some situations feel very complicated and then I have to look to myself and see what energy I have left and what it needs to be used on. Sometimes I go into the battle and other times I capitulate so as to be able to gather myself in preparation for the next battle which will be just around the corner.

'We can't let people go on studying just because they think it is fun!' said the smiling face across the table. I didn't even protest. I had passed all my exams, enough for a BA.

The job centre was not interested in what it had cost me.

Yep, so I am in a 'down' period again. I don't know why. I don't know whether it is physical or psychological, that is just the way it is. It feels like someone has given me a ton of stones to carry around with me. My arms are weak, I can't face anything, all the writing I have done feels wasted, meaningless, idiotic.

I wonder how long I will be like this?

The other night I laughed until I cried when I thought that 'everything is going to get worse – just wait; there are bound to be many ironic catastrophes just around the corner'.

I was almost hysterical with laughter. The odd thing is that I didn't cry as much as previously. In the past I would have cried buckets, but now they barely cover the bottom.

The air has literally gone out of me. I have a puncture in my right tyre.

Threshold episode

Mum and Dad have renovated their bathroom and there is now a slightly higher step in the doorway than before. They have had a wooden ramp made, a threshold eliminator which could be put in place when I visit and otherwise be removed.

This small plan touched a nerve in me. In fact I reacted so strongly that, when at last I decided to tell them what I thought, I couldn't hold back the tears. Having the ramp hidden away is like saying *we will remove every trace of Anne-Pia, deny her, only let it be visible when she, the problem, is here.*

They never intended me to think about it in that way: it was just a practical idea. Once I managed to put into words how their decision made me feel, the ramp has been in place ever since, whether I am there or not.

Frida Bertine had been having some help with her homework for a while. Together we had struggled and had joyous moments with secondary-school maths. Again I felt that I would like to work with pupils who need help. I had laid the idea down ever since that catastrophic doctor's visit. Now I met people who, when I was open with them, encouraged and supported me in doing something of that sort. I had progressed sufficiently with myself that I believed what they said, 'pupils need you, you are a wise soul'.

My heart was thumping in my chest as I sat there with my documents in my hand. Documents which, through a government 'back-to-work' scheme, mean that I can work in a secondary school for ten months. Fill them out and return them.

My head didn't know if I would manage it. Painful comments about me spun round in my head, making my hands sweat and my heart race. My heart was trying to say something different from my head. My heart wanted me to try. Reminded me of the positive comments. Made me remember everything that I can do, everything I have inside me.

In the end my head chose to trust my heart and allowed my hands to sign the papers.

The comment that I had become slimmer came as a surprise. How much weight had I lost? I had no idea as I hadn't weighed myself for a long time. For the first time I realised that I had been through some tough years, and now I could dare to believe that everything will be alright for me. I trained, ate less, my body was better for it and my soul was healing. Why hadn't I done this before? I know the answer; because I have not been emotionally ready for it before now. I had to repair the emotional and psychological parts of me before I could concentrate on the physical side.

In the past I 'needed' the fat to create a barrier between myself and my painful thoughts and feelings. I 'needed' the fat to protect me from the world. I now face the world much stronger and more open. I have convinced myself that I will manage to be slim again, and I have discovered that it doesn't matter if I define myself in a different way to the 'right' way. Yes, there is grief that not everyone can see the me that I really am, but at the same time it gives me space that others don't have. I do not have to be like everyone else – I will never be stereotyped.

It all began with thoughts in my mind when I lay on a mat and looked at myself as a newborn baby. That thought had been there in the meditation group during my A-level years although I didn't know what it was. The same thought that has been in hibernation, and yet at the same time has quietly developed and eventually come out, convincing me that I am allowed to love myself for who I am, not despite it.

I now want what is best for me. Every time I am included and seen for who I really am, my healthy self-image is strengthened. Every gram and kilo that I lose emphasises the way forward. Thoughts like these create a ballast for the times I meet physical hindrances which emphasise my disability and everything I feel is wrong with me. Most important for me is that my healthy identity is so strong that it can lift me up and give me the strength to love myself.

POSTSCRIPT

Travelogue from the *Lord Nelson,* the ship without limitations

In August 2008, Måløy was the host for the Tall Ship Races. After the festivities in Måløy, the ships sailed on to Bergen, where the second leg of the race was to continue on to Holland. One of these ships is unlike all the others, in that it was built with the idea of not having physical limitations. We are two friends with differing handicaps who were so fortunate as to be on board as the only Norwegians on the ship *Lord Nelson* for a week's journey from Måløy to Bergen. It was an experience never to be forgotten, one which I'd like to share with others. The following description is based on my own experiences of the trip.

I will never forget how I celebrated my thirty-first birthday, or where I had been on the preceding days – on board a 130-foot, three-masted English sailing ship lying at a jetty in Bergen together with several other large and small sailing ships. In this fine ship, which for the past week had been home to me and 49 fellow sailors, I was presented with a lemon cake decorated with marshmallows, icing sugar, candles and my name written in red icing. The cake emerged out onto the deck accompanied by a choir of voices singing 'happy birthday to you'. For a few seconds my newly-brown face turned red again. The evening was no anticlimax. Those of us from the *Lord Nelson* paraded, together with all the other crews, through the centre of Bergen, from the Bergenhus fortress, round the Wharf and on to the Market Place where a stage show was in full swing with prize giving, group singing and a performance by a sea-shanty group. From there we went on to a crew party in the Grieg Hall, with food and a dance for 3,000 crew members.

I found myself right in the middle of the Norwegian part of the Tall Ship Races. Not in the competitive part, but the bit called *Cruise in Company*; the graceful leg of the journey in which the ship was able to display itself, and at the same time its crew could experience all the beautiful fjords and mountains along Norway's west coast.

So how did I end up in the midst of all this? Since I have spinal damage and am wheelchair-bound the idea of crewing on a sailing ship was something I had never imagined that I would get to experience. The closest I'd ever got to anything like this was a wet and windy three-hour trip on the *Atløy* around the islands in the West Norway district of Flora, during which I had to spend the entire trip outside on deck because there wasn't room for the wheelchair to fit indoors.

When a friend, Jan Helge Oksholen, rang from Måløy before the summer holidays and asked whether I wanted to travel with one of the ships during the Tall Ship Races, it was this memory that came to mind during the second that I hesitated. I had never heard that, for over twenty years, there have been two English ships, *Lord Nelson* and *Tenacious*, which are the only ships in the world that are entirely accessible for people with disabilities. But when I was asked whether I wanted to join one of these ships, I knew that when life sends a unique chance like this it is impossible to say no. 'There are two available places for this leg of the Tall Ship Races', Jan Helge told me. I was able to take a friend with me, Lene Jordanger, who has MS.

So it was that, on Sunday 3 August 2008, we embarked on *Lord Nelson* as the only Norwegians on board. We were each allocated a *buddy*, a personal assistant to whom we could turn if we needed help with anything. My buddy, Vanessa, a twenty-year-old girl from England, had applied to come on board as a buddy. Her name was put into a hat and from there drawn out to become my buddy for this trip.

The ship has ten permanent crew members as well as forty ordinary crew, of whom half have disabilities. There are no passengers; everyone has to join in and help, working together to get things done and learning from each other.

Vanessa and I soon got on well, which was a good thing because the timetable showed that we were, that very night, to share a two-hour watch from midnight until two before being relieved by Lene and her buddy, Barbara, who were to take the next two hours. As we were still lying at quay in Måløy our job was to ensure that no unauthorised people came on board and that, when our crew returned from shore during the night, they changed their cabin-number labels from *out* to *in* on the registration board.

Monday began with a wake-up call half an hour before breakfast at eight o'clock. Those who had been on early watch had already finished their breakfast shift. Safety on board is important, so one hour later the permanent crew went through the safety procedures with us; the alarm also sounded and we carried out an evacuation practice. This of course meant that I and my evacuation team were shown the correct way to get a wheelchair user up on deck. A strap was to be placed permanently under and round the wheelchair cushion. Then it was just a case of the others fastening me to the block and tackle on the ceiling. This made it simpler to get me up stairs. When there was not an evacuation situation I used the various lifts to get up and down from deck.

Eight of the cabins were designed to have room for a wheelchair beside the bed. The cabins contained bunk beds, on which the buddy took the upper bunk. We had duvets, two pillows and a mattress which was not bad to lie on. A so-called *lee cloth* is a safety guard made of strong fabric fastened with straps to prevent the sleeper from being tipped out of bed during the night. This came in useful later on in the trip, on the one night when we were sailing downwind. On that occasion we really experienced the swaying of the ship, but that was also the night in which I slept best of all the nights on board. This was perhaps because, instead of lying and hearing the even hum of the engine, I had the feeling of lying in a water-bed whilst being gently rocked to sleep. There was only one day of sailing, on account of the wind not being in the right direction or being absent altogether, but we certainly experienced the difference between using the forward motion of the engine and sailing with the wind. Whilst sailing in the wind I helped to hoist the sail right up until I felt I was no longer being responsible and ought to use my energy to stop myself rolling backwards and forwards on the flat deck. In the end I found myself a place on the deck where I simply chained myself securely to something solid. Of course, I could simply have gone below deck but I didn't want to miss out on the atmosphere; how the ship was riding the waves, how the wind was filling the sails, and how the cold crept in under the skin. My fellow sailors brought me coffee and wondered whether they ought to bring me more clothes, but I said that this was not necessary, that I would soon go below deck in any case. All the same I remained fastened there right up until I felt that I'd absorbed enough of the atmosphere to be able to recall it when I got back home. At that point it was time to go down to the bar.

Those of us who were ordinary crew were divided into groups of ten. Together we shared out two four-hour shifts per day. In addition we all had one day in the galley together with one person from each of the other groups. The leader of the watch ensured that we were given the information that she in turn had received from higher authority – the permanent crew – and she also made sure that tasks were shared out internally during watches. When on watch on the bridge we each had a half hour as lookout both to port and starboard (we chose to use the English words as everything else was going on in English) during which we scanned the sea for items in the water that were too small to show up on the radar.

We also steered the ship. The wheel was so easy to manoeuvre that it could be done with two fingers. The compass could be turned to all angles and for those with a visual impairment that was also an audio compass that spoke the ship's course out loud. Since I sat in my own wheelchair, and was therefore too low to watch how the actual ship turned and manoeuvred its way through the Krakhellesundet Sound and the Aurland Fjord, the compass was the only way I could keep in touch with my own steering. Right in the middle of the narrowest part the pilot told me to take my eyes off the compass and just look round for a moment. Around me I saw steep mountainsides, so close that it felt as though I could just reach out with my arm and touch them. It was scary and fascinating at the same time to see how close to land I was navigating the ship and I found it safer to look back and concentrate fully and completely on the compass. Afterwards, the others, who had not been on watch, said that they would never have guessed that it was me, the amateur, who had steered the ship through the narrow sound and that they had been entirely relaxed and at ease.

In Olden we had a surprising offer from the local tourist operatives to visit the Briksdalsbreen Glacier. This was very popular amongst the British and the five Lithuanians. We took a bus up to the café area, after which most people carried on up the glacier on foot. A handful of us drove buggies up to the car park below the glacier.

But this was nevertheless not the high point of that day for me. An important part of the concept of the trip was concerned with investigating and expanding one's personal boundaries. Even before I had ever seen the ship I had heard that it was possible for wheelchair users to get high up the mast. I wasn't entirely sure whether I should take this idea seriously and laughed light-heartedly with the people who had mentioned this possibility. The day before we arrived in Olden, all those who could walk were shown the procedure for climbing the masts. Afterwards the First Officer, Steve, came over and said that the following day there was to be *assisted climbing*, in which we three wheelchair users were to be hoisted up the mast. Many people asked me whether I really dared to do this, but as soon as the idea became real, as soon as there really was a chance, there was no longer any question – I was going to do it! Firstly because I would regret it far more if I didn't try and secondly because coming home and telling people that I'd been there would be something entirely different from saying that I'd watched other people doing it. After all, how many times have I had to sit there, watching other people doing things?

So, the next day, my wheelchair and I were securely fastened in a harness with endless safety ropes and, in a regular rhythm, I was hoisted straight up by ten of my fellow sailors. 105 feet up I was received by two other members of the crew who were standing on a fenced-in platform. There I sat, enjoying the view across Olden, waving to and photographing the people standing in the platform on the other mast, before steady hands lowered me back down to the deck. Only for a second, way up there, had I consciously to remind myself not to think about just how high up I was. The rest of the time I enjoyed 'hanging free', in the secure knowledge that I was in the best of hands.

The weather was good, with a little rain and sunshine alternately. As I mentioned, only once was there enough wind to sail, but even so we were given training about the various sails and how they should be hoisted correctly. The bravest people ventured out onto the yardarm, which is the horizontal mast beam, in order to wrap the sail neatly into itself so that it looked good for arriving in the next harbour. In the little galley, Wendy conjured up the most amazing meals. Every day there was fresh, good, warm and cold food for breakfast, lunch and dinner; a full English breakfast, stews, pies, salmon with rice, banoffee pie, lamb, baked and roasted potatoes and salad. And between meals, time was found for two or three coffee or tea breaks with biscuits and nibbles. In line with old sailing tradition, this type of break was essential so that the crew could get out a pipe and take a smoke, as well as a little coffee. This was called *smoko*, and even today it is *smoko* that is called over the loudspeaker when it's time for a coffee break.

I can't omit mentioning one particular episode that I valued very much. According to the timetable, the Gloppe Fjord (my home fjord) was not supposed to be one of the stops. Early one morning, at four-ish, when I came up onto the bridge to begin my watch I noticed that the surroundings through which we were gliding seemed very familiar. It began to dawn on me that we had just passed the Anda-Lote ferry; two ferry ports that straddle the mouth of the Gloppe Fjord, only seven miles from my home village of Sandane. Naturally, I enthusiastically informed the rest of the watch and the First Officer, Steve, that we were very close to my home. Steve fetched the map and I showed him where Sandane was located. About a day later, whilst I was washing my hair in the disabled bathroom, a message came down from the First Officer that we would be passing Anda-Lote again in another hour and a half, at about 9 o'clock, in case I wanted to let anyone know at home. In the meantime, everyone got ready for the day's *happy hour*, which means an hour of washing, brass-polishing and anything else that needed doing. As we passed Anda we looked to see whether anyone had turned out and, through the binoculars, I could see Dad and Frida, my sister, standing on the rocks by the witches' monument. When told, all the crew who were not too occupied with work, waved, and Steve sounded the ship's hooter. And then we were past, and it was straight back to work polishing the ship's bell. But that the First Officer and crew took the time to do this struck me as a lovely gesture and something that was a fine experience for those on land as well.

When we arrived at Flåm, since there was not room for us at Balestrand after all, there was a treat for us there as well. After a little persuasion and feminine wiles from our Norwegian pilot Solgunn, we were given free tickets for the Flåm Railway. A Mexican ship was also lying at anchor there and after a joint crew party on our ship many people took the opportunity to return with the Mexicans to visit their legendary bar.

To the strains of *God Save the Queen*, followed by cannon salute, *Lord Nelson* arrived in Bergen. I was on kitchen duty but was given permission to go out to witness the arrival. Whilst we in the galley were filling and emptying the dishwasher, drying and stacking and making everything ready for the next meal, Captain Claire was doing a formidable job manoeuvring the ship into position amongst all the others. In the afternoon parade, Lene sat at the front with our banner held high. It was a long way to walk, so she had agreed with Barbara to get a lift in one of the ship's wheelchairs, and I had a push from Vanessa. As the parade route was fairly long, the local arrangers had given us the opportunity to wait until the parade arrived down at the flower market, before we joined in, but I didn't think much of the idea of missing out on the start together with all the others. Vanessa was also almost angry when I translated the suggestion to her, to check that she didn't mind giving me a push. 'They seem to have misunderstood everything this ship is about,' she exclaimed. 'We are here to do everything together, whatever it may be!'

Even though most of the journey had taken place within our own county, and the furthermost point was Bergen which is not so terribly far from home, it felt like returning to Norway when we came ashore from the express boat back in Måløy. A week on an English ship, surrounded by the English language, and with the great admiration and enthusiasm of overseas tourists for the landscape around us, had surrounded us like a bubble and created an illusion about our distance from home.

But even though we had been in familiar territory the whole time, our horizons had been broadened, and new doors opened, because we had experienced the reality that the impossible can well become possible!

NEW BEGINNING

January 2012

Three years have passed since my book was released in Norway.

I have been invited to many different locations to give speeches about my story. I have talked to nurses, physicians, social workers, therapists, politicians, young people, teachers, parents, and fellow handicapped. It has been a joy to find out the similar thoughts and feelings we humans have, in spite of our different backgrounds and challenges, and I am humble when I see someone being touched by words I once never wanted anyone to hear.

A few years earlier I nervously signed the documents to work in an upper school for ten months. It was something new and scary that I didn`t know if I could handle. The school was the one I myself had attended as a teenager, but my worries of becoming a colleague of my old teachers soon disappeared. The pupils were young children, and I was extremely nervous before every class because I got the old feeling of not being good enough, just as I felt as a young kid. It was a really good thing working through my fears like this, though. What I enjoyed the most in this job was working one-to-one with the pupils who needed more attention, just like I had imagined me doing so many years ago. It amazed me to see the change from behaving badly in class to really calming down (well, sometimes relaxing too much!) when we were by ourselves. And they never made a fuss about having a teacher in a wheelchair!

Soon I mainly managed to relax and just enjoy being there with the teenagers; talking, teaching, listening... while thanking my lucky stars I was not a teenager any longer.

During this period I started on a masters degree in *Regional Language and Culture*, the study of the written culture of Norwegian Nynorsk, one of two official written standards for the Norwegian language. After a year I had one more year left. I had all the obligatory exams one must have before getting started on the big written work. Then I stopped. Not because I got sick or I didn`t enjoy it; I had learnt a lot from great teachers in the small group of students. But I had to do a reality check. My ten months in the school was up without any chance of extension. The employment services were amalgamating with the social services and the national insurance office, and the new organisation was renamed NAV (Norwegian labour and welfare organization; see page 183), and I was offered employment experience in the new, local office. This was May of 2009: some months later I was offered a paid job at the office. My first real long-term paid job! By now I had forgotten about the masters degree. A degree that of course would look good on the paper, but which I only started to better my chances of getting a job. Now I had one, I wanted to use my energy on the job.

I started out working 50% of the time, then 70%, then I had to be convinced by both my boss and my boyfriend that I was able to work 100%. They were right; I did manage. My experiences from being on the other side of the table were well worth bringing in to NAV. I wanted to meet people with the same respect I longed to be greeted with when *I* was a client at the job office.

On a more personal note, life has handed me a surprising twist when it called back onto the stage someone who for a short period was very close to me but had been out of my life for years. In the chapter *A new image of her body* he is mentioned briefly but intensely. Since then he had changed his name. He is now called Gus.

I don't like admitting it, but Facebook (my sisters had nagged me for a year to enter Facebook and I had just got a site) was the link to reunite with him. My friend Janne, who went to school in Denmark with me, had got the idea of finding old school mates on Facebook. His name was the first one that popped into my head, and I asked if she had located him. The next day she did, and soon she got a response, and I got a friend request. A couple of months later he called me and we talked like it had been only yesterday since we parted. Then I was going on a one-day trip to Denmark for Christmas with friends where I met up with him. The following month he came to Norway for a visit. When he left it was only to get more of his stuff.

One of the many strengths Gus has is that he knows my situation from the inside because his older brother is also in a wheelchair. So he doesn't care about what others might find unpleasant or strange. He knows what he is getting into, and we can skip a lot of the awkwardness. To my frustration he is not afraid to push me to the limits of what I think I can do, even though I object for whatever it's worth. To be pushed like this is something I am not used to, but I can see that it is making me more aware of what kind of person I want to be. Today Gus and I have bought a small house in the Norwegian forest, 10 km from Nordfjordeid, where we will start our own tree-workshop and where we are going to build a new life together.

Norway has a state-funded healthcare system paid for predominantly through taxes taken directly from salaries. There is no specific health contribution fund. Doctors charge kr180 (Norwegian krone) which is the equivalent of £20 (pounds sterling) for their consultations. Patients pay for their medication up to a maximum amount which varies each year. In 2012 the amount was kr1980 (about £214). When this amount is exceeded patients are entitled to a card which exempts them from fees for the rest of the year.

Ny Arbeids og Velferdsforvaltning (NAV) is the Norwegian Labour and Welfare Organisation. It was established on 1 July 2006, as a merger of three former organisations: The National Insurance Organisation (state), The National Employment Service (state), and The Social Welfare System (municipal). NAV is responsible for the National Insurance Scheme (NIS), a state scheme that guarantees everybody a basic level of welfare such as benefits for illness, accidents, bodily defects, pregnancy, birth, disability, death, and loss of the breadwinner as well as for unemployment and old age. Anyone who is admitted to hospital, and who is a member of the National Insurance Scheme, does not pay for treatment, medication or hospital accommodation.

Since 2002 healthcare policy has been delivered by five health regions plus the municipalities. These regions have their own budgets and are financed through the government. The hospitals provide the public with specialized treatment. In addition, research and training of healthcare personnel is one of four main statutory responsibilities for the health trusts. From 2003 Norwegian citizens have been entitled to choose their hospital. Patients are entitled to access their medical records and be told about the possible risks and side effects of their treatment. Anyone hurt as a result of treatment failure within the health service, has a right to compensation.

The Norwegian Ministry of Health and Care Services determines healthcare policy and oversees the state system. The Helseøkonomiforvaltningen or Norwegian Health Economics Administration (HELFO) is a subordinate institution linked to the Norwegian Directorate of Health since 2009. HELFO provides direct payments to various health service providers, individual reimbursement for certain medicines, dental services and health services abroad and issues The European Health Insurance Card. In addition, it is in charge of the regular GP scheme, which entitles patients to have a regular GP.

Norway has three spinal-cord injury units, located within the best University Hospitals in three regional health authorities. Sunnaas Hospital is based in the south, but for many years received patients from all over Norway, including Anne-Pia. Western Norway Regional Health Authority's unit is at Haukeland Hospital in Bergen, where Anne-Pia has been involved since 2006. Mid Norway Regional's unit is at St Olav Hospital in Trondheim. The three units conduct research, coordinate the rehabilitation process and train and advise patients and relatives.

Beitostolen Health Sports Centre, located in Valdres, was opened in 1970. It was, to a great extent, founded upon the ideas and personal experiences of the blind visionary Erling Stordahl (1923-1994) who served as the director of the centre from its beginning in 1970 until 1994. The programme's concept was established in cooperation with national health authorities. The building of the centre was made possible by means of a national fundraising campaign organised by the Lions Clubs International.

A stay at the centre, usually four weeks for adults and two and a half weeks for children, is financed by the Norwegian Social Security System. The payment covers the expenses of any guides, helpers or parents who are needed for successful participation in the programmes. The short-term stay at the centre is one part of a rehabilitation process – one link in a 'rehabilitation chain'.

Sandane is the village where Anne-Pia grew up. It is the administrative centre of the municipality of Gloppen in Sogn and Fjordane county. Sandane has an area of 2 ¾ square kilometres (600 acres or 0.9 square miles) and, in 2011, had a population of 2,138. Historically Norway is divided into a number of districts which are defined by geographical features like valleys, mountains ranges, and fjords. Many such regions were petty kingdoms up to the early Viking age. Sogn and Fjordane consist of three geographical regions like this: Sogn, Sunnfjord, and Nordfjord (in English Fjordane means *the fjords*). Each of these regions are named after their biggest fjord; The Sogne fjord (largest fjord in Norway, second longest in the world), the Sunn fjord (meaning the fjord in the south) and the Nord fjord (means the fjord in the north) The regional district were Sandane lies is Nordfjord.

Gloppen hotel in Sandane is a member of 'historic hotels' in Norway which is a organization containing many of Norways`s most charming hotels and restaurants. They are required to have quality rooms, service and food. Many guests who visit for salmon fishing in the Gloppe river stay in the hotel. Gloppen is the largest agricultural municipality in this county and the hotel offers local food such as meat, fruit, berries, herbs and potatoes.

Sandane is located at the inland end of the Gloppe fjord, along highway E39, and 20 kilometres (12 miles) south of Nordfjordeid, a village which is the administrative centre of the municipality of Nordfjordeid. Many people from Anne-Pia's village go there for work or shopping. At Nordfjordeid is an opera house and a psychiatric centre (for both adults and children) and, until it was closed recently, the local hospital was situated in Nordfjordeid.

In Norway there are so many fjords that ferries become very important. To go to Nordfjordeid from Sandane, for example, you drive for fifteen minutes to the ferry, load the car on board for the eight-minute journey to Lote, and then have a five-minute drive to the centre of Nordfjordeid.

Anne-Pia's family (her parents still live in the house in which she grew up) live 1 kilometre northwest of the centre of Sandane. A ten-minute drive from the house lies Sandane Airport, Anda. Oslo is one hour away by air, and Bergen only forty minutes; by bus from Sandane it takes seven hours to Oslo and five hours to Bergen.

The Gloppen Ungdomsskole (similar to an English secondary school, which takes students aged 13-15) and Firda Videregående Skole (similar to an English further education college, which takes students aged 16-18) is located in Sandane. There are several elementary or primary Schools around the Gloppe fjord. From Anne-Pia's house it is a fifteen-minute walk uphill to her former primary school, Austrheim. To both Gloppen Primary School and Firda College it is about fifteen to twenty minutes walking, four to five minutes in a car, or for Anne-Pia's eldest brother one minute on a bicycle when you are too late for school every morning!

Anne-Pia's father works with marketing in the local newspaper *Firda Tidend*. When Anne-Pia was little the newspaper was located ten minutes south of Sandane centre. Her Dad still works there, but now the paper has moved to the centre. Anne-Pia's Mum ended up working with the elderly in the Gloppen care centre for most of her life; she only worked with infants when she lived in Bergen.

Anne-Pia's eldest brother Paul is working with satellites and computers in the military establishment in Honefoss, her younger brother, Peter, is a dentist in Bergen. Her sisters, Guro and Constanse, also live in Bergen. Guro trained as a nurse and is now a student, and Constanse was educated in healthcare and is now studying as a dental hygienist. The youngest sister Frida Bertine is studying media in Lillehammer.